THE
LOGIC OF VEGETARIANISM

ESSAYS AND DIALOGUES

BY

HENRY S. SALT

AUTHOR OF
"ANIMALS' RIGHTS, CONSIDERED IN RELATION TO SOCIAL
PROGRESS"

THE MORALIST AT THE SHAMBLES.

Where slaughter'd beasts lie quivering, pile on pile,
And bare-armed fleshers, bathed in bloody dew,
Ply hard their ghastly trade, and hack and hew,
And mock sweet Mercy's name, yet loathe the while
The lot that chains them to this service vile,
Their hands in hideous carnage to imbrue:
Lo, there!—the preacher of the Good and True,
The Moral Man, with sanctimonious smile!
"Thrice happy beasts," he murmurs, "'tis our love,
Our thoughtful love that sends ye to the knife
 (Nay, doubt not, as ye welter in your gore!);
For thus alone ye earned the boon of life,
And thus alone the Moralist may prove
His sympathetic soul—by eating more."

PREFACE

In preparing this "Logic of Vegetarianism" for a new edition, I have carefully re-read a sheaf of press opinions which greeted the first appearance of the book some seven years ago, with the hope of profiting by any adverse criticism which might point out arguments that I had overlooked. In this, however, I have been disappointed, for, apart from a few such objections as that raised in all seriousness by the *Spectator*—that I had not done justice to the great problem of what would become of the Esquimaux—the only definite complaint which I can find is that the representatives of flesh-eating whom I have introduced in the dialogues are deliberately made to talk nonsense. "It is easy," said one critic, "to confute an opponent if you have the selection of the arguments and the framing of the replies."

I ought not, perhaps, to have expected that the assurance given in my introductory chapter (p. 2) as to the authenticity of the anti-vegetarian pleadings would shield me from this charge; indeed, the *Vegetarian Messenger*, in a friendly review of the book, expressed doubt as to the policy of using dialogue at all, because, as it remarked, "the arguments against vegetarianism are often so silly that it looks as if the author had set up a man of straw in order to demolish him." Yet, as the *Messenger* itself added, "there is not an argument against vegetarianism quoted in this volume which we have not, time after time, seen seriously brought forward by our opponents." Surely it would be a strange thing if food reformers had to avoid any terse presentment of their adversaries' reasoning for the very fact of its imbecility!

And there is this further question. If I have failed to include in my selection the effective arguments against vegetarianism, where and what are they? Looking through those cited in the press notices, I can discover none that seem to be formidable; but rather than again be suspected of unfair suppression, let me frankly quote the following specimens of the beef-eater's philosophy:

> "The proof that man should eat meat is that he always has done so, does now, and always will."

And again:

> "Nobody will want to make out that he (the advocate of vegetarianism) is wrong, but folk will just go on suiting themselves as before. Shelley and Thoreau, Wagner and Edward FitzGerald, were vegetarians, but, then, Wellington and Gladstone partook of the roast beef of Old England, and were none the worse."

There is a sublime simplicity about these statements which is most impressive, but I cannot think that any wrong is done to the case against vegetarianism by not including them in a discussion which purports to be a logical one.

H. S. S.

CONTENTS

THE
LOGIC OF VEGETARIANISM

INTRODUCTORY

It is the special purpose of this book to set forth in a clear and rational manner the logic of vegetarianism. To the ethical, the scientific, and the economic aspects of the system much attention has already been given by well-accredited writers, but there has not as yet been any organised effort to present the *logical* view— that is, the dialectical scope of the arguments, offensive and defensive, on which the case for vegetarianism is founded. I am aware that mere logic is not in itself a matter of first-rate importance, and that a great humane principal, based on true natural instinct, will in the long-run have fulfilment, whatever wordy battles may rage around it for a time; nevertheless, there is no better method of hastening that result than to set the issues before the public in a plain and unmistakable light. I wish, therefore, in this work, to show what vegetarianism is, and (a scarcely less essential point) what vegetarianism is *not*.

For though, owing to the propaganda carried on for the last fifty years, there has been an increasing talk of vegetarianism, and a considerable discussion of its doctrines, there are still very numerous misunderstandings of its real aims and meaning. In this, as in other phases of the great progressive movement of which vegetarianism is a part, to give expression to a new idea is to excite a host of blind and angry prejudices. The champions of the old are too disdainful to take counsel with the champions of the new; hence they commonly attribute to them designs quite different from those which they really entertain, and unconsciously set up a straw man for the pleasure of pummelling him with criticism. Devoid always of a sense of sympathy, and mostly of a sense of humour, they absurdly exaggerate the least vital points in their adversaries' reasoning, while they often fail to note what is the very core of the controversy. It is therefore of great concern to vegetarianism that its case should be so stated as to preclude all possibility of doubt as to the real issues involved. If agreement is beyond our reach, let us at least ascertain the precise point of our disagreement.

With a view to this result, it will be convenient to have recourse now and then to the form of dialogue, so as to bring into sharper contrast the *pros* and *cons* of the argument. Nor will these conversations be altogether imaginary, for, to avoid any suspicion of burlesquing the counter-case of our opponents by a fanciful presentment, I shall introduce only such objections to vegetarianism as have actually been insisted on—the stock-objections, in fact, which crop up again and again in all colloquies on food reform—with sometimes the very words of the flesh-eating disputant. It is not my fault if some of these objections appear to be foolish. I have often marvelled at the reckless way in which those who would combat new and unfamiliar notions step forth to the encounter, unprovided with intellectual safeguards, and trusting wholly to certain ancient generic fallacies, which, if we may judge from their appearance in all ages and climates, are indigenous in the human mind. Many of the difficulties which the flesh-eater to-day propounds to the vegetarian are the same, *mutatis mutandis*, as those which have at various times been cast in the teeth of the reformer by the apologists of every cruel and iniquitous custom, from slave-holding to the suttee.

To show the unreality of these sophisms, by clearing away the misconceptions upon which they rest, and to state the creed of vegetarianism as preached and practised by its friends rather than as misapprehended by its foes—such is the object of this work. To make "conversions," in the ordinary sense, is not my concern. What we have to do is to discover who are flesh-eaters by ingrained conviction, and who by thoughtlessness and ignorance, and to bring over to our side from the latter class those who are naturally allied to us, though by accident ranged in opposition. And this, once more, can only be done by making the issues unmistakable.

Incidentally, I hope these pages may suggest to our antagonists that vegetarians, perhaps, are not the weak brainless sentimentalists that they are so often depicted. It is, to say the least of it, entertaining when a critic who has just been inquiring (for example) "what would become of the animals" if mankind were to desist from eating them, goes on to remark of vegetarians that "their hearts are better than their heads." Alas, we cannot truthfully return the compliment by saying of such a philosopher that his head is better than his heart! It cannot be too strongly stated that the appeal of vegetarianism, as of all humane systems, is not to heart alone, nor to brain alone, but to brain and heart combined, and that if its claims fail to win this double judgment they are necessarily void and invalid. The test of logic, no less than the test of feeling, is deliberately challenged by us; for it is only by those who can think as well as feel, and feel as well as think, that the diet question, or indeed any great social question, can ever be brought to its solution.

WHY "VEGETARIAN"?

The term "vegetarian," as applied to those who abstain from all flesh food, but not necessarily from such animal products as eggs, milk, and cheese, appears to have come into existence over fifty years ago, at the time of the founding of the Vegetarian Society in 1847. Until that date no special name had been appropriated for the reformed diet system, which was usually known as the "Pythagorean" or "vegetable diet," as may be seen by a reference to the writings of that period. Presumably, it was felt that when the movement grew in volume, and was about to enter on a new phase, with an organised propaganda, it was advisable to coin for it an original and distinctive title. Whether, from this point of view, the name "vegetarian" was wisely or unwisely chosen is a question on which there has been some difference of opinion among food reformers themselves, and it is possible that adverse criticism would have been still more strongly expressed but for the fact that no better title has been forthcoming.

On the whole, the name "vegetarian" seems to be fairly serviceable, its disadvantage being that it gives occasion for sophistry on the part of captious opponents. In all controversies such as that of which vegetarianism is the subject there are verbalists who cannot see beyond the outer shell of a word to the thing which the word signifies, and who delight to chop logic and raise small obstacles, as thus:

VERBALIST: Why "vegetarian"?

VEGETARIAN: Why not "vegetarian"?

VERBALIST: How can it be consistent with vegetarianism to consume, as you admit you do, milk, butter, cheese, and eggs, all of which are choice foods from the animal kingdom?

VEGETARIAN: That entirely depends on what is meant by "vegetarianism."

VERBALIST: Well, surely its meaning is obvious—a diet of vegetables only, with no particle of animal substance.

VEGETARIAN: As a matter of fact, such is not, and has never been, its accepted meaning. The question was often debated in the early years of the Vegetarian Society, and it was always held that the use of eggs and milk was *not* prohibited. "To induce habits of abstinence from the flesh of animals (fish, flesh, fowl) as food" was the avowed aim of vegetarianism, as officially stated on the title-page of its journal.

VERBALIST: But the word "vegetarian"—what other meaning can it have than that which I have attributed to it?

VEGETARIAN: Presumably those who invented the word were the best judges of its meaning, and what they meant by it is proved beyond a doubt by the usage of the Society.

VERBALIST: But had they a right thus to twist the word from its natural derivation?

VEGETARIAN: If you appeal to etymology, that raises another question altogether, and here, too, you will find the authorities against you. No one has a better right to speak on this matter than Professor J. E. B. Mayor, the great Latin scholar, and he states that, looking at the word etymologically, "vegetarian" cannot mean "an eater of vegetables." It is derived from *vegetus*, "vigorous," and means, strictly interpreted, "one who aims at vigour." Mind, I am not saying that the originators of the term "vegetarian" had this meaning in view, but merely that the etymological sense of the word does not favour your contention any more than the historical.

VERBALIST: Well, what *does* "vegetarian" mean, then? How do you explain it yourself?

VEGETARIAN: A "vegetarian" is one who abstains from eating the flesh of animals, and whose food is *mainly* derived from the vegetable kingdom.

The above dialogue will show the absurdity and injustice of charging vegetarians, as the late Sir Henry Thompson did, with "equivocal terms, evasion—in short, untruthfulness," because they retain a title which was originally invented for their case. The statement that vegetarians have *changed* the meaning of their name, owing to inability to find adequate nourishment on purely vegetable diet, is founded on similar ignorance of the facts. Here are two specimens of Sir Henry Thompson's inaccuracy. In 1885 he wrote:

> "It is high time that we should be spared the obscure language, or rather the inaccurate statement, to which milk and egg consumers are committed, in assuming a title which has for centuries belonged to that not inconsiderable body of persons whose habits of life confer the right to use it."[1]

Observe that Sir Henry Thompson was then under the impression that the name "vegetarian" (invented in 1847) was "centuries" old! Nor, names apart, was he any more accurate as regards the practice itself, for it can be proved on the authority of a long succession of writers, from the time of Ovid to the time of Shelley, that the use of milk and its products has been from the first regarded as compatible with the Pythagorean or "vegetable" diet. The fact that some individual abstainers from flesh have also abstained from all animal substances is no justification of the attempt to impose such stricter abstinence on all vegetarians on peril of being deprived of their name.

Thirteen years later Sir Henry Thompson's argument was entirely changed. His assertion of the *antiquity* of the name "vegetarian" was quietly dropped; in fact, its *novelty* was now rather insisted on.

> "They (the "vegetarians") emphatically state that they no longer rely for their diet on the produce of the vegetable kingdom, differing from those who originally adopted the name at a date by no means remote."[2]

But our critic was again absolutely mistaken. There is no difference whatever between the diet of those who adopted the name at the date by no means remote and that of those who bear it now. Now, as then, there are some few vegetarians who abjure all that is of the animal, but the rule of the Society now, as then, is that the use of eggs and milk is permissible. At the third annual meeting, held in 1850, it was stated by one of the speakers that "the limits within which the dietary of the Vegetarian Society was restricted excluded nothing but the flesh and blood of animals."

To avoid any possible misunderstanding, let me repeat that it is no part of the case for vegetarianism to defend the *name* "vegetarian" in itself; it may be a good name or a bad one. What we defend is our right to the title, an indefeasible historical claim which is not to be upset by any such unfounded and self-contradictory assertions as those quoted.

But it may be said that even if the title is historically genuine, it would be better to change it, as it evidently leads to misunderstanding. We should be perfectly willing to do this, but for two difficulties: first, that no other satisfactory title has ever been suggested, and secondly that, as the word "vegetarian" has now a recognised place in the language, it would scarcely be possible to get rid of it; at any rate, the substitute, to have the least chance of success, would have to be very terse, popular, and expressive. Take, for example, the name "flesh-abstainer," or "akreophagist," proposed by Sir Henry Thompson. The obvious objection to such terms is that they are merely *negative*, and give the notion that we are abstinents and nothing more. We do not at all object to the use of the term "flesh-abstainer" as explanatory of "vegetarian," but we do object to it as a substitute, for as such it would give undue prominence to our disuse of flesh food, which, after all, is merely one particular result of a general habit of mind. Let us state it in this way: Our view of life is such that flesh-eating is abhorrent and impossible to us; but the mere fact that this abstinence attracts the special attention of flesh-eaters, and becomes the immediate subject of controversy, does not make it the sum and substance of our creed. We hold that in a rational and humanised society there could be no question at all about such a practice as flesh-eating; the very idea of it would be insufferable. Therefore we object to be labelled with a negative term which only marks our divergence from other persons' diet; we prefer something that is positive and indicative of our own. And until we find some more appropriate title, we intend to make the best of what we have got.

The whole "Why 'vegetarian'?" argument is, in fact, a disingenuous one. The practical issue between "vegetarians" and flesh-eaters has always been perfectly clear to those who wished to understand it, and the attempt made by the verbalists to distract attention from the *thing* in order to fasten it on the *name* is nothing but sophistical. Of this main practical issue, and of the further distinction between the "vegetarian" or flesh-abstaining diet and the purely vegetable diet, I will speak in the following chapter.

THE *RAISON D'ÊTRE* OF VEGETARIANISM

Behind the mere name of the reformed diet, whatever name be employed (and, as we have seen, "vegetarian" at present holds the field), lies the far more important reality. What is the *raison d'être*, the real purport of vegetarianism? Certainly not any *a priori* assumption that all animal substances, as such, are unfit for human food; for though it is quite probable that the movement will ultimately lead us to the disuse of animal products, vegetarianism is not primarily based on any such hard-and-fast formula, but on the conviction, suggested in the first place by instinctive feeling, but confirmed by reason and experience, that there are certain grave evils inseparable from the practice of flesh-eating. The aversion to flesh food is not chemical, but moral, social, hygienic. Believing as we do that the grosser forms of diet not only cause a vast amount of unnecessary suffering to the animals, but also react most injuriously on the health and morals of mankind, we advocate their gradual discontinuance; and so long as this protest is successfully launched, the mere name by which it is called is a matter of minor concern. But here on this practical issue, as before on the nominal issue, we come into conflict with the superior person who, with a smile of supercilious compassion, cannot see *why* we poor ascetics should thus afflict ourselves without cause.

SUPERIOR PERSON: But why, my dear sir—why should you refuse a slice of roast beef? What is the difference between roasting an ox and boiling an egg? In the latter case you are eating an animal in embryo—that is all.

VEGETARIAN: Do you not draw any distinction between the lower and the higher organisation?

SUPERIOR PERSON: None whatever. They are chemically identical in substance.

VEGETARIAN: Possibly; but we were talking, not of chemistry, but of morals, and an egg is certainly not morally identical with an ox.

SUPERIOR PERSON: How or where does the moral phase of food-taking enter the science of dietetics?

VEGETARIAN: At a good many points, I think. One of them is the question of cannibalism. Allow me to read you a passage from the "Encyclopædia Britannica": "Man being by nature {?} carnivorous as well as frugivorous, and human flesh being not unfit for human food, the question arises why mankind generally have not only avoided it, but have looked with horror on exceptional individuals and races addicted to cannibalism. It is evident on consideration that both emotional and religious motives must have contributed to bring about this prevailing state of mind."

SUPERIOR PERSON: Of course. Why read me all that?

VEGETARIAN: To show you that what you call "the moral phase of food-taking" has undoubtedly affected our diet. The very thought of eating human flesh is revolting to you. Yet human flesh is chemically identical with animal flesh, and if it be true that to boil an egg is the same thing as to roast an ox, it follows that to butcher an ox is the same thing as to murder a man. Such is the logical position in which you have placed yourself by ignoring the fact that all life is not *equally* valuable, but that the higher the life the greater the responsibility incurred by those who destroy it.

Or it may be that the superior person, instead of denying that morals affect dietetics, himself poses as so austere a moralist as to scorn the wretched half-measure of merely abstaining from flesh food while still using animal products. The result is in either case the same. The all-or-nothing argument is sometimes put forward in this fashion:

SUPERIOR PERSON: Well, as far as the right or wrong of the question is concerned, I would not care to be a vegetarian at all, unless I were a thorough one. What can be the good of forswearing animal food in one form if you take it in another?

VEGETARIAN: But surely it is rational to deal with the worst abuses first. To insist on an all-or-nothing policy would be fatal to any reform whatsoever. Improvements never come in the mass, but always by instalment; and it is only reactionists who deny that half a loaf is better than no bread.

SUPERIOR PERSON: But in this case I understand that it is quite possible to be consistent. There are individuals, are there not, who live upon a purely vegetable diet, without using milk or eggs? Now, those are the people whose action one can at least appreciate and respect.

VEGETARIAN: Quite so. We fully admit that they are in advance of their fellows. We regard them as pioneers, who are now anticipating a future phase of our movement.

SUPERIOR PERSON: You admit, then, that this extreme vegetarianism is the more ideal diet?

VEGETARIAN: Yes. To do more than you have undertaken to do is a mark of signal merit; but no discredit attaches on that account to those who have done what they undertook. We hold that "the first step," as Tolstoy has expressed it, is to clear one's self of all complicity in the horrible business of the slaughter-house.

SUPERIOR PERSON: Well, I must repeat that, were I to practise any form of asceticism, I should incline to that which does not do things by halves.

VEGETARIAN: Of course. That is invariably the sentiment of those who do not do things at all.

Asceticism! such is the strange idea with which, in many minds, our principles are associated. It would be impossible to take a more erroneous view of modern vegetarianism; and it is only through constitutional or deliberate blindness to the meaning of the movement that such a misconception can arise. How can we convey to our flesh-eating friends, in polite yet sufficiently forcible language, that their diet is an abomination to us, and that our "abstinence," far from being ascetic, is much more nearly allied to the joy that never palls? Is the farmer an ascetic because, looking over into his evil-smelling pigsty, he has no inclination to swill himself from the same trough as the swine? And why, then, should it be counted asceticism on our part to refuse, on precisely the same grounds, to eat the swine themselves? No; our opponents must clearly recognise, if they wish to form any correct notion of vegetarianism, that it is based, not on asceticism, but æstheticism; not on the mortification, but the gratification of the higher pleasures.

We conclude, then, that the cause which vegetarians have at heart is the outcome, not of some barren academic formula, but of a practical reasoned conviction that flesh food, especially butchers' meat, is a harmful and barbarous diet. Into the details of this belief we need not at present enter; it has been sufficient here to show that such belief exists, and that the good people who can see in vegetarianism nothing but a whimsical "fad" have altogether failed to grasp its true purport and significance. The *raison d'être* of vegetarianism is the growing sense that flesh-eating is a cruel, disgusting, unwholesome, and wasteful practice, and that it behoves humane and rational persons, disregarding the common cant about "consistency" and "all-or-nothing," to reform their diet to what extent and with what speed they can.

THE PAST AND PRESENT OF VEGETARIANISM

But, it may be said, before entering on a consideration of this reformed diet, for which such great merits are claimed by its exponents, the practical man is justified in asking for certain solid assurances, since busy people cannot be expected to give their time to speculations which, however beautiful in themselves, may prove at the end to be in conflict with the hard facts of life. And the first of these questions is, What is the historic basis of vegetarianism? In what sense is it an old movement, and in what sense a new one? Has it a past which may serve in some measure to explain its present and guarantee its future?

Such questions have been dealt with fully from time to time in vegetarian literature.[3] I can here do no more than epitomise the answers. Vegetarianism, regarded simply as a practice and without relation to any principle, is of immemorial date; it was, in fact, as physiology shows us, the original diet of mankind, while, as history shows us, it has always been the diet of the many, as flesh food has been the diet of the few, and even to this day it is the main support of the greater part of the world's inhabitants. Numberless instances might be quoted in proof of these assertions; it is sufficient to refer to the people of India, China, and Japan, the Egyptian fellah, the Bedouin Arab, the peasantry of Russia and Turkey, the labourers and miners of Chili and other South American States; and, to come nearer home, the great bulk of the country folk in Western Europe and Great Britain. The peasant, here and all the world over, has been, and still is, in the main a vegetarian, and must for the most part continue so; and the fact that this diet has been the result, not of choice, but of necessity, does not lessen the significance of its perfect sufficiency to maintain those who do the hard work of the world. Side by side with the tendency of the wealthier classes to indulge more and more in flesh food has been the undisputed admission that for the workers such luxuries were unneeded.

During the last half-century, however, as we all know, the unhealthy and crowded civilisation of great industrial centres has produced among the urban populations of Europe a craving for flesh food, which has resulted in their being fed largely on cheap butchers' meat and offal; while there has grown up a corresponding belief that we must look almost entirely to a flesh diet for bodily and mental vigour. It is in protest against this comparatively new demand for flesh as a necessity of life that vegetarianism, as a modern organised movement, has arisen.

Secondly, if we look back for examples of deliberate abstinence from flesh—that is, of vegetarianism practised as a *principle* before it was denoted by a name—we find no lack of them in the history of religious and moral systems and individual lives. Such abstinence was an essential feature in the teaching of Buddha and Pythagoras and is still practised in the East on religious and ceremonial grounds by Brahmins and Buddhists. It was inculcated in the humanitarian writings of great "pagan" philosophers, such as Plutarch and Porphyry, whose ethical precepts, as far as the treatment of the lower animals is concerned, are still far in advance of modern Christian sentiment. Again, in the prescribed regimen of certain religious Orders, such as Benedictines, Trappists, and Carthusians, we have further unquestionable evidence of the disuse of flesh food, though in such cases the reason for the abstinence is ascetic rather than humane. When we turn to the biographies of individuals, we learn that there have been numerous examples of what is now called "vegetarianism"—not always consistent, indeed, or continuous in practice, yet sufficiently so to prove the entire possibility of the diet, and to remove it from the category of generous aspiration into that of accomplished fact.[4]

But granting that there is historic basis for the vegetarian system, the question is asked whether, on ethnological evidence, it does not appear that the dominant races have been for the most part carnivorous, and the subject races vegetarian—a line of argument which always appeals strongly to the patriotic Briton.

> PATRIOT: Come, now; it is all very well to talk of philosophers and poets, and I have no doubt you can point to such names among the founders of your creed, but what I ask is, Were the founders of the British Empire vegetarians? Were any great empires ever founded by vegetarians? Was Julius Cæsar a vegetarian? Was Wellington a vegetarian? Can you give me any instance of vegetarianism as a fighting force?

> VEGETARIAN: As regards the rank and file of conquering armies, there are many such instances, both in ancient and modern history. The diet of the Roman soldier was not that of a flesh-eater, and the Roman Empire was assuredly not won by virtue of flesh-eating, but by the hardihood which

could subsist on simple rations of wheat, oil, and wine. So, too, the armies which built up the earlier empires of Egypt and Assyria were, for the most part, vegetarian. That is to say, while the rulers and wealthy classes of fighting nations have been carnivorous, the bulk of the soldiery, drawn from the frugal peasant class, has been unaccustomed to such luxuries. The idea that the flesh-eating races have everywhere subjugated the vegetarians is quite illusory.

PATRIOT: But surely in India the flesh-eating Mohammedan has always conquered the vegetarian Hindu?

VEGETARIAN: Not by any means always. It took him centuries of fierce fighting to do so, with all the advantages of religious fanaticism on his side, as against an enemy weakened by internal dissension and an enervating climate. But that Mohammedanism does not depend on flesh food for its fighting qualities may be seen from the case of that special ally and favourite of yours, the Turk. Let me read you what the *Standard* said of him some twenty years back: "From the day of his irruption into Europe, the Turk has always proved himself to be endowed with singularly strong vitality and energy. As a member of a warlike race, he is without equal in Europe in health and hardiness. He can live and fight when soldiers of any other nationality would starve. His excellent physique, his simple habits, his abstinence from intoxicating liquors, and his normal vegetarian diet, enable him to support the greatest hardships, and to subsist on the scantiest and simplest food." Have I said enough to show you that vegetarianism *may* be a fighting force?

It will be objected, perhaps, that when food reformers claim these fighting qualities for their diet they are proving just a little too much for their principles, as, for example, in the reference to the sanguinary Turk as a practical vegetarian. If the outcome of vegetarian diet is to be war and massacre, how is the system any better than that which it fain would supersede? This brings us back to the starting-point of the present chapter, the distinction between what may be called the old and the new vegetarianism. We have seen that, so far as the common practice is concerned, abstinence from flesh food is as old as history itself, and that rarer instances may be cited of practice and principle combined; but when we regard vegetarianism as a propagandist movement, a conscious endeavour to benefit not merely the individual man, but human society itself, we have to recognise that it is a *new* movement. From a mere habit of the many, or piety of the few, it has become a reasoned principle, an organised system, with a name and nomenclature of its own: in vulgar language, it is an *-ism*, and, like other kindred *-isms*, a part of the great humanitarian impulse of the past hundred years.

The significance of this distinction is considerable. Modern "vegetarianism" is the same, yet not the same, as the "flesh abstinence" that dates from earlier times—the same in so far as the actual dietary is concerned, and in some fewer cases the same in principle, but different altogether in the spirit by which that principle is informed; and for this reason it would be ridiculous to judge vegetarianism as a whole by the character of those races who happen to have been abstainers from flesh, and who are merely quoted as proving the physical sufficiency of the diet. In a word, ethnical vegetarianism and ethical vegetarianism are two very different things.

It has also to be remembered that the modern vegetarian appeals not to humane instinct only, but to physiological facts, and that the movement has now become to a very large extent a scientific and hygienic one, thus again differing widely from the merely empirical and unconscious vegetarianism of earlier times. These several aspects of the system will be reviewed in succeeding chapters; it is enough here to repeat that vegetarianism as a practice is immemorial, as a precept is of great antiquity, but as an organised cult is one of the new revolutionary forces of modern times.

STRUCTURAL EVIDENCE

We have seen, then, that vegetarianism, though new as a propagandist doctrine, has its historical record; but if we wish thoroughly to understand its origin, we must go back beyond history to the more ancient and more durable evidence of the organic structure of Man. Here we come in conflict with what is, perhaps, the strangest of the many strange prejudices that oppose the humane diet—the superstition, so common among the uneducated, and connived at, if not shared, by some of the "scientific" themselves, that the verdict of comparative anatomy is fatal to the vegetarian claims. So far is this from being the case that the great naturalists, from Linnæus onward, give implicit judgment to the contrary, by classing mankind with the frugivorous family of the anthropoid apes. Thus Sir Richard Owen says:

> "The apes and monkeys, which man most nearly resembles in his dentition, derive their staple food from fruits, grain, the kernels of nuts, and other forms in which the most sapid and nutritious tissues of the vegetable kingdom are elaborated; and the close resemblance between the quadrumanous and the human dentition shows that man was, from the beginning more especially adapted 'to eat of the fruit of the trees of the garden.'"[5]

And here is the more recent verdict of Sir Benjamin Richardson:

"On the whole, I am bound to give judgment on the evidence of the teeth rather in favour of the vegetarian argument. It seems fairest of fair to read from nature that the teeth of man were destined—or fitted, if the word destined is objected to—for a plant or vegetable diet, and that the modification due to animal food, by which some change has been made, is practically an accident or necessity, which would soon be rectified if the conditions were rendered favourable to a return to the primitive state.... By weighing the facts that now lie before us, the inference is justified that, in spite of the very long time during which man has been subjected to an animal diet, he retains in preponderance his original and natural taste for an innocent diet derived from the first-fruits of the earth."[6]

Yet, in spite of such testimony, and more of an equally authoritative kind, it is quite a common thing for some flesh-eating "scientist" to allege against vegetarianism the conformation of the human teeth or stomach.

SCIENTIST: But our teeth, my good friend, our teeth! What can be the use of your talking about vegetarianism, when we both of us carry in our mouths a proof of the necessity of flesh-eating.

VEGETARIAN: But surely you do not hold the popular fallacy that man's canine teeth class him among the carnivora?

SCIENTIST: They prove at least that he is an eater of flesh as well as of vegetables. Why else has he got such teeth?

VEGETARIAN: Why has a gorilla got such teeth? "For the purpose of combat and defence," Owen tells us, not of food. And if a gorilla, with "canines" much more developed than man's, is a frugivorous animal, why must man with less developed "canines" be carnivorous?

SCIENTIST: Well, well; let us turn to the digestive organs, then. Look at the immense difference between the human stomach and that of the true herbivora. How can mankind get the required nutriment from herbs, when we have not the necessary apparatus for doing so?

VEGETARIAN: But it has never been argued by us, nor is it in any way essential to our argument, that mankind is *herbivorous*. What have the herbivora to do with the question?

SCIENTIST: I have seen them quoted in your books as instances of strength and endurance——

VEGETARIAN: To dispel the illusion that there is no chemical nutriment in anything but flesh food; but that is quite a different thing from asserting that man is himself herbivorous. The point at issue is simple. You charge vegetarians with flying in the face of Nature. We show you, from your own authorities, that the structural evidence, whatever that may be worth (it was you who first appealed to it), pronounces man to have been originally neither carnivorous, nor herbivorous, but *frugivorous*. If you think otherwise, what do you make of the apes?

The close similarity that exists between the structure of man and that of the anthropoid apes is the hard fact that cannot be evaded by the apologists of flesh-eating. In the conformation alike of brain, of hands, of teeth, of salivary glands, of stomach, we have indisputable proof of the frugivorous origin of man—indeed, it is not seriously questioned by any recognised authority, that man was a fruit-eater in the early stages of his development. As far as comparative anatomy throws light on the diet question, mankind and the apes are, so to speak, "in the same box," and he who would disprove the frugivorous nature of man, must also disprove the frugivorous nature of the anthropoid apes, a predicament of which the more intelligent of our opponents are keenly aware. And this brings us to the second branch of the subject of this chapter.

Whatever his original structure, it is argued, man has extended his resources in the matter of food, and has long been "omnivorous," while his middle position between the carnivora and herbivora indicates that he is naturally suited for a "mixed diet." *Omnivorous*, it will be noted, is the blessed word that is to bring comfort to flesh-eaters, and the inconvenient apes, whom the naturalists class as frugivorous, have somehow to be dragged in under the category of "omnivorous." But, first, a word about the meaning of this saving term.

Now, I wish to make it plain that vegetarians are not wedded to any *a priori* theory that the lines of dietetic development are stringently limited by the original structure of man. If the flesh-eater appeals, as he so often does, to physical structure, with the intent of attributing carnivorous instincts to mankind, we confront him with an array of scientific opinion which quickly makes him wish he had let the subject alone; and if he insists on the "evolutional" rather than the "natural" aspect of the problem, we are equally ready to meet him on this newer ground. But we decline to fall victims to the rather disingenuous quibble that lurks in the specious application to mankind of the term "omnivorous."

For what, in the present connection, does the word "omnivorous" mean? It cannot, obviously, mean that man should, like the hog, eat *everything*, for, if so, it would sanction not only flesh-eating, but cannibalism, and we should have to class mankind (so Professor Mayor has wittily remarked) as *hominivorous*! It must mean, presumably, that man is fitted to eat not *everything*, but *anything*— vegetable food or animal food—implying that he is eclectic in his diet, free to choose what is good and reject what is bad, without being bound by any original law of nature.[7] To the name "omnivorous," used not in the hoggish sense, but in this rational sense, and not excluding, as the scientists would absurdly make it exclude, the force of *moral* and other considerations, the vegetarian need raise no objection. Man is "omnivorous," is he? He may select his own diet from the vegetable and animal kingdoms? Well and good: that is just what we have always advised him to do, and we are prepared to give reasons, moral and hygienic, why, in making the selection, he should omit the use, not of all animal products, but of flesh. The scientists cannot have it *both* ways. They cannot dogmatise on diet as a thing settled by comparative anatomy, and *also* assert that man is "omnivorous"—*i.e.*, free to choose what is best.

But let us return to our monkeys.

SCIENTIST: You just now quoted the gorilla as a frugivorous animal, but, on further consideration, I cannot admit him to be so. He is omnivorous—like man. I have Sir Richard Owen's authority for it.

VEGETARIAN: What! Does the ape rush upon the antelopes, and rend them with those canine teeth of his? How horrible!

SCIENTIST: Not exactly that; but it was stated by Sir Henry Thompson that "Sally," the large chimpanzee once so popular in the Zoological Gardens, was not infrequently supplied with animal food.

VEGETARIAN: Well, and how does that prove that the chimpanzee is not naturally frugivorous? I should imagine that any one of us, if placed in a cage, and stared at all the year round by a throng of gaping visitors, might be liable to aberrations. Even a vegetarian might do the same.

SCIENTIST: But in their wild state also the baboons are known to prey on lizards, young birds, eggs, etc., when they can get them. Perhaps you were not aware of this when you called the apes frugivorous?

VEGETARIAN: I was quite aware of it, and in view of the exceedingly small importance of these casual pilferings as compared with their staple diet, I maintain that they *are*, for all practical purposes, frugivorous. Indeed, so far from this mischievous penchant of the apes being an argument against vegetarianism, it is most suggestive as explaining how the early savages may have passed, almost by accident at first, from a frugivorous to a mixed diet.

SCIENTIST: Well, at any rate, it indicates that apes have a tendency to become omnivorous.

VEGETARIAN: Yes, if you like to express it so; and it is still more evident that men have that tendency. But the question is whether the tendency is rightly interpreted as giving a sanction to *flesh-eating*. For flesh-eating, as we use the term, means the breeding, destroying, and devouring of highly-organised mammals, and is a very different thing from the egg and lizard hunting in which the monkeys sometimes indulge. If you would confine your flesh-eating to a few insects and nestlings, you would have a better right to quote the example of the apes.

Has flesh-eating been a necessary step in man's progress? Without access to the flesh-pots, it has been asked, would not the race have remained in the groves with the orangs and the gorillas? I do not see that vegetarians need concern themselves to answer such speculations, which, interesting though they are, do not bear closely on the present issue. For though, as we have seen, the testimony of the past is in favour of a frugivorous origin, the problem of the present is one which we are free to solve without prejudice, and whether the past use of flesh food, by a portion of the world's inhabitants, has helped or hindered the true development of man is a matter for individual judgment. We may have our own opinion about it. But what we are concerned to prove is that flesh-eating can offer no advantages to us *now*.

THE APPEAL TO NATURE

Of the many dense prejudices through which, as through a snowdrift, vegetarianism has to plough its way before it can emerge into the field of free discussion, there is none perhaps more inveterate than the common appeal to "Nature." A typical instance of the remarkable misuse of logic which characterises such argument may be seen in the anecdote related by Benjamin Franklin, in his "Autobiography," of the incident which induced him to return, after years of abstinence, to a flesh diet. He was watching some companions sea-fishing, and observing that some of the fish caught by them had swallowed other fish, he concluded that, "If you eat one another, I don't see why we may not eat you"—a confusion of ichthyology and morals which is ludicrous enough as narrated by Franklin, but not essentially more foolish than the attempt so frequently made by flesh-eaters to shuffle their personal responsibility on to some supposed "natural law."

But let the carnivorous anthropologist speak for himself:

ANTHROPOLOGIST: Now, understand me! I think this vegetarianism is well enough as a sentiment; I fully appreciate your aspiration. But you have overlooked the fact that it is contrary to the laws of Nature. It is beautiful in theory, but impossible in practice.

VEGETARIAN: Indeed! That puts me in an awkward position, as I have been practising it for twenty years.

ANTHROPOLOGIST: It is not the individual that I am speaking of, but the race. A man may practise it perhaps; but mankind cannot do so with impunity.

VEGETARIAN: And why?

ANTHROPOLOGIST: Because, as the poet says, "Nature is one with rapine." It is natural to kill. Do you dare to impugn Nature?

VEGETARIAN: Not at all. What I dare to impugn is your incorrect description of Nature. There is a great deal more in Nature than rapine and slaughter.

ANTHROPOLOGIST: What? Do not the beasts and birds prey on one another? Do not the big fish eat the little fish? Is it not all one universal struggle for existence, one internecine strife?

VEGETARIAN: No; that is just what it is not. There are *two* principles at work in Nature—the law of competition and the law of mutual aid. There are carnivorous animals and non-carnivorous, predatory races and sociable races; and the vital question is—to which does man belong? You obscure the issue by these vague and meaningless appeals to the "laws of Nature," when, in the first place, you are quoting only part of Nature's ordinance, and, secondly, have not yourself the least intention of conforming even to that part.

ANTHROPOLOGIST: I beg your pardon. In what do I not conform to Nature?

VEGETARIAN: Well, are you in favour of cannibalism, let us say, or the promiscuous intercourse of the sexes?

ANTHROPOLOGIST: Good gracious, my dear sir! I must entreat you——

VEGETARIAN: Exactly! You are horrified at the mere mention of such things. Yet these habits are as easily justified as flesh-eating, if you take "Nature" as your model, without specifying *whose* nature? The nature of the conger and the dog-fish, or the nature of civilised man? Pray tell me *that*, Mr. Anthropologist, and then our conversation may not be wholly irrelevant.

The idea that the Darwinian doctrine of the "struggle of life" justifies any barbarous treatment of inferior races is ridiculed by so distinguished an authority as Prince Kropotkin, who points out that Darwin does *not* teach this. "He proves that there is a struggle for existence in order to put a check on the inordinate increase of species. But this struggle is not to be understood in a crude and exclusive sense; there is a law of competition, but there is also—what is still more important—a law of mutual aid, and as soon as the scientist leaves his laboratory, and comes out into the open woods and meadows, he sees the importance of this law. Only those animals who are mutually helpful are really fitted to survive; it is not the strong, but the co-operative species that endure."[8] So, too, with reference to the strange notion that a guide for human conduct may be deduced from some particular animal instinct, taken at haphazard from its surroundings, a timely warning is addressed to such crude reasoners by Professor J. Arthur Thomson: "What we must protest against is that one-sided interpretation, according to which individualistic competition is Nature's sole method of progress.... The precise nature of the means employed and ends attained must be carefully considered, when we seek from the records of animal evolution support or justification for human conduct."[9]

It may be said, however, that though man is fitted to co-operate peacefully with his fellows, he is not bound by any such ties of brotherhood to the lower animals, and that it is "natural" that he should prey on the non-human races, even if it be not natural that he should seek pleasure at the cost of his fellow-man. But, in reality, Nature knows no such bridgeless gulf between the human and the non-human intelligence; and it is impossible, in the light of modern science, to draw any such absolute line of demarcation between man and "the animals" as in the now discredited theory of Descartes. We are learning to get rid of these "anthropocentric" delusions, which, as has been pointed out by Mr. E. P. Evans, "treat man as a being essentially different and inseparably set apart from all other sentient creatures, to which he is bound by no ties of mental affinity or moral obligation"; whereas, in fact, "man is as truly a part and product of Nature as any other animal, and this attempt to set him up as an isolated point outside of it is philosophically false and morally pernicious."[10]

The talk, then, about Nature being "one with rapine" is a mere form of special pleading, which will not stand examination in the full light of fact. If man is determined to play the part of tiger among his less powerful fellow-beings, he will have to go elsewhere than to Nature to obtain a warrant for his deeds, for as far as the indications of Nature carry weight, they suggest that man, by his physical structure and his compassionate instincts, belongs unmistakably to the sociable, and not the predatory tribes; and that by constituting himself a "beast of prey" on a vast artificial scale, he is doing the greatest possible wrong to nature (*i.e.*, to *his own* nature) instead of conforming to it. Our innate horror of bloodshed—a horror which only long custom can deaden, and which, in spite of past centuries of violence, is so powerful at the present time—is proof that we are not naturally adapted for a sanguinary diet; and, as has often been pointed out, it is only by delegating to others the detested work of slaughter, and by employing cookery to conceal the uncongenial truth, that thoughtful persons can tolerate the practice of flesh-eating. If Nature pointed us to such a diet, we should feel the same instinctive appetite for raw flesh as we now feel for ripe fruit, and a slaughter-house would be more delightful to us than an orchard. It is not Nature, but custom, that is the guardian deity of the flesh-eater.

25

But we have not quite exhausted the appeal to Nature; we have still to speak of the common objection to vegetarianism that "it is necessary to take life."

ANTHROPOLOGIST: I have a most important argument to put before you. Must you not face the fact that, in this imperfect world, it is necessary to take life? How can it be immoral to do what necessity imposes?

VEGETARIAN: We do not say that it is immoral to "take life," but that it is immoral to take life *unnecessarily*. It is not immoral, for instance, to destroy rats and mice, because it is necessary to do so. It *is* immoral to kill animals for the table, because it is *not* necessary to do so. Did you ever tread on a beetle?

ANTHROPOLOGIST: Yes, by accident. I could not help it. I am a most humane man.

VEGETARIAN: Of course. But supposing that you wished to murder someone, would you think yourself justified in doing so because you had trodden on beetles—because, in fact, sometimes it is "necessary to take life?"

ANTHROPOLOGIST: Certainly not. How can you suspect me of being so immoral? There is a great difference between taking the life of a beetle by accident and of a man by design. There are *degrees* of responsibility, you know.

VEGETARIAN: Ah! you have got your answer, then.

How is it, we wonder, that rational beings can commit themselves to such irrational arguments as this appeal to what is called "Nature" but is in reality only an isolated section of Nature, viewed apart from the rest? Let Benjamin Franklin himself supply the answer. For in narrating that incident of the cod-fish to which I have alluded, he humorously hints that his philosophical conclusion, "If you eat one another, I don't see why we may not eat you," was not uninfluenced by the fact that he had been "a great lover of fish" in early life, and that the fish smelt "admirably well" as it came out of the frying-pan; and he sagely adds that one of the advantages to man of being a "reasonable creature" is that he can find or make a "reason" for anything he has a mind to do. Such is the logic of the flesh-eater, in which the wish is father to the thought, and mixed thinking leads by a convenient process to a mixed diet.

THE HUMANITARIAN ARGUMENT

It will have been noted that the anti-vegetarian arguments which have so far come under review have been mainly such as are based on purely *materialistic* grounds, as if the question were wholly one for doctors and scientists to decide; and it has been shown that, even thus, there is no sort of warrant for the supercilious dismissal of vegetarianism as a theory condemned in advance by some superior tribunal. But the question is not one for the *ipse dixit* of the specialist. It is also a moral question of very great moment, and this fact gives a new significance to such unwilling admissions as that made by the *British Medical Journal*, that "man can obtain from vegetables the nutriment necessary for his maintenance in health"—*i.e.*, from vegetables only, much more, therefore, from a vegetable diet with the addition of eggs and milk. The practicability of vegetarianism being thus fully granted, it is impossible to pretend that moral considerations are not relevant to the controversy, and that in forming an opinion on the vexed problem of diet we should not give due weight to the promptings of humaneness.

People often talk as if the humanitarian plea were some fanciful external sentiment that has been illogically thrust into the discussion; whereas in truth it is one of the innermost facts of the situation which no sophistry can escape. Our humane instincts are unalterably implanted in us, and we cannot deny them if we would; to be *human* is to be *humane*. "There is something in human nature," says an old writer,[11] "resulting from our very make and constitution, which renders us obnoxious to the pains of others, causes us to sympathise with them, and almost comprehends us in their case. It is grievous to see or hear (and almost to hear of) any man, or even any animal whatever, in torture." And now that modern science has demonstrated the close kinship that exists between human and non-human, the greater is the repulsion that we feel at any wanton ill-usage of animals.

This is now so generally admitted that the point in dispute is not so much the duty of humaneness, as some particular application of that duty, as in the present case to the slaughter of animals for food. What have humane people to say to the tremendous mass of animal suffering inflicted, in the interests of the table, on highly-organised and sensitive animals closely allied to mankind? By the unthinking, of course, these sufferings, being invisible, are almost wholly overlooked, while the deadening power of habit prevents many kindly persons from exercising, where their daily "beef" and "mutton" are concerned, the very sympathies which they so keenly manifest elsewhere; yet it can hardly be doubted that, if the veil of custom could be lifted, and if a clear knowledge of what is involved in "butchery" could be brought home, with a sense of personal responsibility, to everyone who eats flesh, the attitude of society towards the vegetarian movement would be very different from what it is now. If it be true that "hunger is the best sauce," it may also be said that the *bon vivant's* most indispensable sauce is *ignorance*—ignorance of the horrible and revolting circumstances under which his juicy steak or dainty cutlet has been prepared.

> BON VIVANT: What is this? "Vegetarian" you call yourself?
>
> VEGETARIAN: And you? You are a *bon vivant*. You "live well," I understand.

BON VIVANT: Not ashamed of enjoying a good dinner, but not greedy, I hope.

VEGETARIAN: Nor cruel, I suppose?

BON VIVANT: Cruel! I subscribe regularly to the Society for the Prevention of Cruelty to Animals.

VEGETARIAN: And *eat* them.

BON VIVANT: Why not? A speedy painless death is no cruelty, is it?

VEGETARIAN: While you are finishing that choice beef steak, I will tell you something of the speedy painless death of steak-producing animals. It may serve as an aid to digestion, like a musical accompaniment.

BON VIVANT: Oh, you won't spoil my digestion. Fire away!

VEGETARIAN: Let us suppose, then, that our friend (on your plate there) hails from Ireland, and at one of the fair grounds, of which there are several thousand in that island paradise, he meets the first agent in his euthanasia—the drover. "On such occasions," says the Report of the late Departmental Committee on the Inland Transit of Cattle, "animals already, perhaps, exhausted and foot-sore from a walk of many miles, stand for hours on the hard road, bewildered by the beating they receive and their unaccustomed surroundings.... It was repeatedly asserted by responsible witnesses that many of the drovers are brutally harsh." So ferocious is the treatment that in many cases, when the animals are slaughtered, the hide, as butchers testify, simply falls off the back, and is worthless even for use as leather. I hope your steak is nice and tender?

BON VIVANT: But why are not the brutal drovers punished for it?

VEGETARIAN: Perhaps because it is not for themselves that they are driving. Then there is the journey in the railway-trucks, and we learn on good authority (Report of the Liverpool S.P.C.A.) that "the animals have frequently gone twenty to twenty-four hours without food at the time they are driven on the boats." As for the delights of the sea-transit, you have read, I suppose, of what happens in cattle-ships?

BON VIVANT: Well, of course, in stormy weather there may be accidents——

VEGETARIAN: No, I am speaking of the ordinary scenes of the cattle traffic, and say nothing of the occasions (not so rare, either) when the boats come into port with blood pouring from their scuppers——

BON VIVANT: Thank you, thank you! that is enough!

VEGETARIAN: We find it stated, in the Report of the Committee of Inquiry into the Irish Cattle Transit, that "the damage sustained by cattle is very serious, and that the principal portion of that damage is due to their treatment during shipment, while on shipboard, and on debarkation." On landing there is more thrashing and tail-twisting, another railway journey, and then—the slaughterman. You have visited a slaughter-house, of course?

BON VIVANT: No, really, I must protest——

VEGETARIAN: Ah, then it should interest you! The drover's task accomplished, the butcher's begins. Yard by yard and foot by foot, with chains fastened to his horns and sharp goads applied to his flanks, the struggling animal is dragged into the dark, blood-stained shed, where he is lucky indeed if he be killed by the first blow of the pole-axe——

BON VIVANT: Shameful! I do not believe you. It cannot be.

VEGETARIAN: Then many well-known eye-witnesses must have strangely perjured themselves. Dr. Dembo, for example, says: "Cases in which several blows are required are very frequent. On my first visit to the Deptford slaughtering yards I found that the number of blows struck was five and more," and he goes on to describe a case which he saw in London, when *twelve minutes* elapsed before the animal——

BON VIVANT: Stop! I will hear no more.

VEGETARIAN: You will hear no more—but will you *eat* more? It is on *you*, not on the brutal drover or slaughterman, that the responsibility falls. For this is the "speedy and painless" way in which animals must be slaughtered that *you* may live well.

"I will hear no more." That, said or implied, is the most common and the most insuperable argument by which the vegetarian is confronted. It is the one great stronghold of flesh-eating which remains from age to age impregnable. For how can even truth convince the deaf and the blind? The horrors of the journey by sea and journey by rail, of the savage drover's goad and the clumsy butcher's pole-axe—if the ordinary man and woman, unimaginative and unfeeling though they are, could see or even hear of these things, the end of the controversy would be nearer. By the few flesh-eaters who have made inquiry, accidental or conscientious, into the facts of the cattle traffic and butchering trade, it is not denied that fearful cruelties are committed. Thus the *Meat Trades Journal*, which is not a sentimental paper, remarks of the sea and land transit, that "our cattle, sheep, and pigs are carried by sea and rail with the minimum care and maximum cost; they are bundled and shunted about as if they were iron."[12] Again, Dr. T. P. Smith, writing in opposition to vegetarianism, allows that the indictment of the slaughter-house "hits a grievous blot on our much-vaunted civilization."[13] There is a mass of printed testimony to the same effect, which can be confirmed, as often as confirmation is needed, by a visit to the shambles. But that is a visit which the ordinary man will neither undertake himself nor hear of from the mouths of others.

Much also might be said of certain special cruelties, such as those involved in the supply of white veal or *pâté de foie gras*, and other so-called delicacies; but it is unnecessary to dwell on such refinements of torture, because it is the ordinary every-day aspects of flesh-eating that are here under debate. It is a terrible fact that the very prevalence of the habit serves, more than anything else, to conceal its full import; and thus a large number of people, who, in any other department of life, would indignantly refuse to profit by the cruel usage of animals, are (without knowing, or at least without recognising it) dependent for their daily food on the continued and systematic infliction of sufferings which, in their magnitude and frequency, surpass all other cruelties whatsoever of which animals are the victims.

These horrors, as I have said, are not realised by those who are personally responsible for them. Or, rather, they are not *directly* realised; for indirectly it is evident enough that the more sensitive conscience of mankind is far from easy about the morality of butchering, and would show still greater uneasiness but for the quieting assurance that flesh food is a strict necessity of existence. This sense of compunction has found at least partial expression in many non-vegetarian works, as, for example, in Michelet's "Bible of Humanity." "Life—death! The daily murder which feeding upon animals implies—those hard and bitter problems sternly placed themselves before my mind. Miserable contradiction! Let us hope that there may be another globe in which the base, the cruel fatalities of this one may be spared to us!"

Now, in view of these facts and these feelings, we have a right to press the advocates of flesh-eating for some more explicit and coherent statement than they have hitherto accorded us of their attitude towards the ethics of the diet question. If, as the scientists themselves admit, there is no such "cruel fatality" as that which Michelet pictured, and if flesh-eating is not to be regarded as necessary, but only as expedient, then it is in the highest degree unreasonable to rule out *humane* considerations from their due share in the settlement of this many-sided problem. The *British Medical Journal* has said that "there is not a shadow of doubt that the use of animals for food involves a vast amount of pain." The same paper has said that "man can obtain from vegetables the nutriment necessary for his maintenance in health." Can it be doubted, that if the average Englishman were made aware of these two facts, he would at least think vegetarianism worthy of a serious trial? To ask, as a superior person of science has asked (not merely in these dialogues, but in actual debate), "How or where does the moral phase of food-taking enter the science of dietetics?" or to take refuge in the common saying that "one man's food is another man's poison," is simply irrelevant. For diet, like other social questions, has its moral aspect, which claims no less and no more than its due importance; and it is because the "scientific" antagonists of vegetarianism have overlooked this fact that their judgments have hitherto been so warped, illogical, and unscientific.

PALLIATIONS AND SOPHISTRIES

It is instructive to note the desperate shifts and subterfuges to which our antagonists have recourse when they find themselves face to face with the humanitarian impeachment of the slaughter-house. If one-half of the popular prejudices were true, it might be supposed that, in the discussion of so "fanciful" and "Utopian" a theory as vegetarianism it would be its supporters who would take refuge in metaphysical quibblings and sophistries, while its opponents would hold sternly to the hard facts of life. But no! for when butchery is the theme we find the exact opposite to be the case, and it is the flesh-eaters, those level-headed deriders of the sentimental, who suddenly became enamoured of the imaginary *what-might-be* and the hypothetical *what-would-otherwise-have-been*, and are disposed to turn their attention to anything rather than to the unpalatable *what-is*.

Now, when the apologists of any form of cruelty are reduced to the plea that it is "no worse" than some *other* barbarous habit, the presumption is that they are in a very bad plight indeed. Yet we frequently hear it said that the fate of animals slaughtered for the table is "no worse" than that of other animals—those perhaps that are used for purposes of draught or burden—a quite pointless comparison, because, even if the statement be true, the one act of injustice can obviously be no excuse for the other. Or it may be that the mortality of man himself, and his liability to disease and accident, are alleged in mysterious justification of his carnivorous habits, the suffering of the animals being represented as brief and momentary in contrast with the pathetic human death-bed—an argument which reached its culminating point in Mr. W. T. Stead's delightful assertion that of all kinds of death he would himself prefer "the mode in which pigs are killed at Chicago," which mode, as he incautiously let out, he did *not* go to see when he visited that city. I do not think we need further discuss such remarkable preference; it will be time enough to do so when we hear of Mr. Stead's lamented self-immolation in the Chicago pig-shambles.

But it is said that domesticated animals owe a deep debt of gratitude to mankind (only to be repaid in the form of beef and mutton), because, by being brought within the peaceful fold of civilisation, they have been spared all the harrowing fears and anxieties of their wild natural life. This, however, is a fallacy to which the great naturalists give no sort of sanction; for it is obvious that, though the life of a wild animal is liable to more sudden perils than that of our tame "livestock," it is not on that account a less happy one, but, on the contrary, is spent throughout in a manner more conducive to the highest health and happiness. Thus, Dr. Alfred Russel Wallace says: "The poet's picture of nature red in tooth and claw, is a picture the evil of which is read into it by our imagination, the reality being made up of full and happy lives, usually terminated by the quickest and least painful of deaths." And Mr. W. H. Hudson: "I take it that in the lower animals misery can result from two causes only—restraint and disease—consequently, that animals in a state of nature are not miserable. They are not hindered or held back.... As to disease, it is so rare in wild animals, or in a large majority of cases so quickly proves fatal, that, compared with what we call disease in our own species, it is practically non-existent. The 'struggle for existence,' in so far as animals in a state of nature are concerned, is a metaphorical struggle; and the strife, short and sharp, which is so common in nature, is not misery, although it results in pain, since it is pain that kills or is soon out-lived."

Let us proceed, then, to the great sophistical paradox that it is better for the animals themselves to be bred and slaughtered than not to be bred at all—that most comfortable doctrine which of late years has been a veritable city of refuge, or grand old umbrella, to the conscientious flesh-eater under stress of the vegetarian bombardment. Hither flock the members of the learned professions, academies, and ethical societies, and fortify their souls anew with this subtle metaphysic of the larder.

> SOPHIST: Of all the arguments for vegetarianism, none, in my opinion, is so weak as the argument from humanity. The pig has a stronger interest than anyone in the demand for bacon.

> VEGETARIAN: Indeed? And is that the view the pig himself takes of it?

> SOPHIST: It is the view *I* take of it, speaking in the interests of the pig. For where would the pig be if we did not eat pork? He would be non-existent; he would be no pig at all.

> VEGETARIAN: And would he be any the *worse* for that?

> SOPHIST: Yes, for he would lose the joy of life. And not the pig alone, but all animals that are bred for human food. Their death is the little price they necessarily pay for the inestimable boon of existence.

> VEGETARIAN: Now, let me first point out to you that it is not only flesh-eating that would be justified by this argument. Vivisection, pigeon-shooting, slavery, cannibalism, any treatment whatsoever of animals or of mankind where they are specially bred for the purpose, might be similarly shown to be a kindness. Do you really mean that?

> SOPHIST: I assume, of course, that the life is a happy one, and the death as painless as possible.

VEGETARIAN: Neither of which conditions is in reality fulfilled! For the wretched creatures that are bred and fed for the shambles have none of the true joys of life, but from the first are mere animated beef, pork, and mutton, while their death is nothing better than a prolonged and clumsy massacre.

SOPHIST: But it need not be so. It is a mere question of police and proper supervision. It should be imperative on all those who confer life on animals to ensure absolute painlessness for the last moment.

VEGETARIAN: It "*should* be"! So it seems that this remarkable kindness of yours is, by your own showing, not an actual but a hypothetical benefit. The animals fulfil their part of the compact by being killed and eaten, and you *might* fulfil your part by killing them painlessly—only you *don't*! Are you serious in talking this stuff?

SOPHIST: This "stuff"? Let me remind you, sir, that I have the authority of such eminent philosophers as Sir Henry Thompson, Mr. Leslie Stephen, Professor D. G. Ritchie, and Dr. Stanton Coit. Do you call their academical reasoning "stuff"?

VEGETARIAN: What else can it be called? For, as a matter of fact, quite apart from the conditions, good or bad, under which the animals live and die, it is a pure fallacy to say that it is a *kindness* to bring them into existence.

SOPHIST: How so, if life is pleasant?

VEGETARIAN: Because it is impossible to compare existence with non-existence. Existence may, or may not, be pleasant; but non-existence is neither pleasant nor unpleasant—it is nothing at all. It cannot, therefore, be an *advantage* to be born, though, when once you *are* born, the good and the evil are comparable. The whole question is a post-natal, not a prenatal one; it begins at birth.

SOPHIST: Well, but supposing you were an animal, would you not prefer——

VEGETARIAN: Oh, that is a very old question. You will find it all in Hansard. It was asked by Sir Herbert Maxwell when he defended the sport of pigeon-shooting in the Debates of 1883. "He wanted to ask the hon. member whether, if he were a blue-rock, he would rather accept life under the condition of his life being a short and happy one, and violently terminated, or whether he would reject life at all upon such terms."

SOPHIST: Hear, hear! That is just what I say.

VEGETARIAN: Then you had better think over Mr. W. E. Forster's reply, which puts the case in a nut-shell. He said that Sir Herbert Maxwell "made one very amusing appeal, by asking him [the member who introduced the Bill] to put himself in the position of a blue-rock. But this would be difficult, for the position was not a blue-rock in existence, but a blue-rock before it was born." Whereat the House laughed, and sophistry was for the moment disconcerted.

But for the moment only; for there have since sprung up many other professors of this metaphysic of the larder, though none of them, with the exception of Dr. Stanton Coit, have had the hardihood to expound their theory in detail—a wise reticence, perhaps, when it is seen how Dr. Coit fared in his conscientious but humourless essay on "The Bringing of Sentient Beings into Existence."

"If the motive," he opined, "that might produce the greatest number of the happiest cattle would be the eating of beef, then beef-eating, so far, must be commended. And while, heretofore, the motive has not been for the sake of cattle, it is conceivable that, if vegetarian convictions should spread much further, love for cattle would (if it be not psychologically incompatible) blend with the love of beef in the minds of the opponents of vegetarianism. With deeper insight, new and higher motives may replace or supplement old ones, and perpetuate but ennoble ancient practices."[14]

The "Ox in a Tea-cup," be it observed, may henceforth become the emblem of the concentrated humanity of the ethical societies!

"But we frankly admit," continues Dr. Coit, "that it is a question whether the love of cattle, intensified to the imaginative point of individual affection for each separate beast, would not destroy the pleasure of eating beef, and render this time-honoured custom psychologically impossible. *We surmise that bereaved affection at the death of a dear creature would destroy the flavour.*"[15]

What a picture is conjured up by the sentence I have italicised—the bereaved moralist, knife and fork in hand, swayed in different directions by the call of duty and the scruples of affection! And then Dr. Coit goes on to express a fear that mankind, if they adopted vegetarianism, might become "less powerful in thought"! I respectfully submit that, in view of the arguments quoted, there is not the smallest possibility of *that*.

The plea that animals might be killed painlessly is a very common one with flesh-eaters, but it must be pointed out that *what-might-be* can afford no exemption from moral responsibility for *what-is*. By all means let us reform the system of butchery as far as it can be reformed—that is, by the total abolition of those foul dens of torture known as "private slaughter-houses," and by the substitution of municipal abattoirs, equipped with the best modern appliances, and under efficient supervision; for there is no doubt that the sum of animal suffering may thus be greatly lessened. There will be no opposition from the vegetarian side to such reform as this; indeed, it is in a large measure through the personal efforts of vegetarians that the subject has attracted attention, whereas the very people who make this prospective improvement an excuse for their present flesh diet are seldom observed to be doing anything practical to carry it into effect. But when all is said and done, it remains true that the reform of the slaughter-house is at best a palliative, a temporary measure which will mitigate, but cannot possibly amend, the horrors of butchery; for it is but too evident that, under our complex civilisation, when the town is so far aloof from the country, and pastoralism can only be carried on in districts remote from the busy crowded centres, it is impossible to transport and slaughter vast numbers of large and highly-sensitive animals in a really humane manner. More barbarous, or less barbarous, such slaughtering may undoubtedly be, according to the methods employed, but the "humane" slaughtering, so much bepraised of the sophist, is an impossibility in fact and a contradiction in terms.

THE CONSISTENCY TRICK

It is certain, then, that the practice of flesh-eating involves a vast amount of cruelty—a fact which cannot be lessened or evaded by any quibbling subterfuges. But, before we pass on to another phase of the food question, we must deal more fully with that very common method of argument (alluded to in an earlier chapter) which may be called the Consistency Trick—akin to that known in common parlance as the *tu quoque*, or "you're another"—the device of setting up an arbitrary standard of "consistency," and then demonstrating that the vegetarian himself, judged by that standard, is as "inconsistent" as other persons. Whether we plead guilty or not guilty to this ingenious indictment depends altogether on the meaning assigned to the term "consistency."

For, as anyone who tries to do practical work in the world will rapidly discover, there is a true and there is a false ideal of consistency. To pretend that in our complex modern society, where responsibilities are so closely interwoven, it is possible for any individual to cultivate "a perfect character," and stand like a Sir Galahad above his fellows—this is the false ideal of consistency which it is the first business of a genuine reformer to put aside; for no human being can do any solid work without frequently convicting himself of inconsistencies when consistency is stereotyped into a formula. On the other hand, there is a true duty of consistency, which regards the spirit rather than the letter, and prompts us not to grasp foolishly at the ideal, like a child crying for the moon, but to push steadily *towards* the ideal by a faithful adherence to the right line of reform, and by ever keeping in view the just proportion and relative value of all moral actions. Let it be remembered that it is this latter consistency alone that has any interest for the vegetarian. His purpose is not to exhibit himself as a spotless Sir Galahad of food reformers, but to take certain practical steps towards the humanising of our barbarous diet system.

Herein will be found the answer to a class of questions frequently put to vegetarians, as to how they find it "consistent with their principles" to use this or that form of food or animal substance. It depends entirely on what their principles are. If their aspirations were of the Sir Galahad order, some of the "posers" would indeed be formidable; but as they do *not* aim at moral perfection, but merely at rational progress, the charge of inconsistency hurtles somewhat harmlessly over their heads. But here let the consistency man have his say:

CONSISTENCY MAN: But what I want to know is this—how you can think it consistent to use milk and eggs?

VEGETARIAN: Consistent with what?

CONSISTENCY MAN: Why, with your own principles, of course.

VEGETARIAN: Or do you mean with your idea of my principles? The two things are not always identical, you know.

CONSISTENCY MAN: You condemn flesh-eating because of the suffering it causes, but it seems to have escaped your notice that the use of milk and eggs is also responsible for much. It is strange that it has never occurred to you——

VEGETARIAN: My good sir, it has occurred to us years and years ago. The question is as old as the movement itself. The cock-and-bull argument, I presume?

CONSISTENCY MAN: I ask, what would become of the cockerels and bull-calves under a vegetarian *régime*? At present your supply of milk and eggs is easy enough, because the young males are killed and eaten by us carnivorous sinners. But are you not, to a certain extent, participators in the deed?

VEGETARIAN: Yes, frankly, to a certain extent (a very limited extent) I think we are. We are content to get rid of the worst evils first.

CONSISTENCY MAN: But is one sort of killing worse than another?

VEGETARIAN: Immeasurably worse. Even if it were necessary under the vegetarian system, to destroy some of the calves at birth, as the superfluous young of domestic animals are now destroyed, it would be ridiculous to compare such restricted killing of new-born creatures with the present wholesale butchery of full-grown and highly-sentient animals in the slaughter-house.

CONSISTENCY MAN: You say "if" it were necessary, but is there any doubt of it?

VEGETARIAN: It is not by any means so certain as you suppose that the slaughter of calves would be unavoidable. Vegetarians use milk sparingly—far more so than flesh-eaters—and a limited amount of milk is obtainable without killing the calf. Nor is there any reason, as Professor Newman has pointed out, why a number of oxen should not be employed as formerly in working the land. But I do not wish to take refuge in future possibilities. I prefer to take the bull-calf argument "by the horns," and admit that, under present conditions, we are indirectly responsible. Call it inconsistency, if you like. If it be inconsistency not to postpone the abolition of the greater cruelties until we also abolish the minor ones, we are willing to be called inconsistent.

It may be noted, in passing, that the zeal with which flesh-eaters urge this counter-charge of "inconsistency" is designed, unconsciously perhaps, to hide an important admission—viz., that where eggs and milk are used there is no necessity for butchers' meat, or, in other words, that vegetarianism is a perfectly feasible diet. "Eggs and milk," says Dr. T. P. Smith, when objecting to their use by vegetarians, "contain a much larger quantity of nutritive material than an equal amount of meat, for which, therefore, they may easily serve as substitutes."[16] If this be granted, the rest is a mere battle of words.

But the cock-and-bull argument, with which may be linked the objection to the use of leather, is only one of many departments of the consistency trick. Another favourite method of convicting vegetarians of inconsistency is to start from the false assumption that vegetarianism is the same thing as Brahminism, and that any destruction of even the lowliest forms of life is therefore reprehensible. "As for the argument based on the cruelty of slaughter-houses," says Mr. W. T. Stead, "I don't see that it bears upon the question, unless you take the extreme Hindoo doctrine as to the wickedness of taking sentient life, even in the shape of lice and adders." That is to say, the terrible and quite unnecessary cruelties inflicted on the most highly-organised and harmless animals in the cattle-ship and slaughter-house do not even "bear upon" the morality of diet, unless we also abstain from killing the most noxious and lowly-organised forms! Of the same nature is the foolish "when-you-drink-a-glass-of-water" fallacy, which argues that, as we necessarily swallow minute organisms in drinking, we need have no scruples as to the needless butchery of a cow or a sheep. The savages who in the good old times used to eat their grandfathers and grandmothers might have justified their dietetic habits on precisely similar grounds.

Nor is it only insects and "vermin" on whose behalf the consistency man is concerned, for plants also have life, and therefore if the vegetarian holds that "it is immoral to take life" (which he does *not*), he must be inconsistent in eating vegetables. As an instance of a common but strange misunderstanding of the vegetarian principle on this subject, I must here quote a passage from the "Science Jottings" of Dr. Andrew Wilson. Note the triumphant tone of the unscientific scientist as he rushes to his absurd conclusion:

> "I have not yet finished with the food faddist. Suppose I find a vegetarian who, more consistent than the run of his fellows, will not touch, taste, nor handle milk, eggs, cheese, or any animal product whatever. I think it is still possible to show him that he is infringing the code he lives by, in so far as its pretensions with the sacredness of life are concerned. Plants, no less than animals, are living things. Their tissues contain living protoplasm, which is the essential physical basis of life everywhere.... I am afraid that the consistent vegetarian must no longer kill a cabbage if he is to live up to the standard of morals he sets up as a kind of fetish in his diet regulations; and to lay low the lettuce, or pluck the apple from its bough, is really a direct infringement of the code which maintains that you have no right to kill any living thing for food. Really this is a monstrous doctrine when all is said and done."[17]

It *is* a monstrous doctrine; and what are we to think of a man of science who attributes such absurdities to vegetarians, and thereupon holds them up to public contempt as inconsistent, when by making inquiry he might at once have learnt that the blunder was on his own side? Once more, then, be it stated that it is not the mere "taking of life," but the taking of life *unnecessarily* that the vegetarian deprecates, and that no criticism of vegetarianism can be of any relevance if it ignores the fact that all forms of life are not of equal value, but that the higher the sensibility of the animal, and the closer his affinity to ourselves, the stronger his claim on our humaneness.

Before leaving this question of "consistency," as affected by the *gradations* of our duty of humaneness to animals, a few words may be said on the practice of fish-eating. It was humorously suggested by Sir Henry Thompson, who, as I have proved in the second chapter of this work, wrote in complete ignorance of the facts and dates of the vegetarian movement, that, as vegetarians have "added" milk and eggs to their diet since their society was founded (a statement quite devoid of truth), they may perhaps still further enlarge their dietary so as to include fish. Here, again, Sir H. Thompson only showed his unfamiliarity with the subject, for his novel proposition was in fact an old one, which has been debated and rejected by the Vegetarian Society in its adherence to its original rule of excluding fish, flesh, and fowl, and nothing else, from its dietary. So far, then, as organised vegetarianism is concerned, those who eat fish are not within the pale of membership; but looked at from the purely *humane* standpoint, it must be admitted that there is an immense difference between flesh-eating and fish-eating, and that those unattached food reformers, not few in number, who for humane reasons abstain from flesh, but feel justified in eating fish, hold a perfectly intelligible position. And I would further note that the very fact of there having been some disposition, wise or unwise, within the vegetarian ranks to recognise the comparative harmlessness of fish-eating, corroborates what I have asserted throughout—that the *raison d'être* of vegetarianism has not been a pedantic hard-and-fast crusade against "animal" substances, but a practical desire to abolish the horrors of the slaughter-house.

This, then, is our parting word to the professors of the Consistency Trick. If they had charged us with the *real* inconsistency—that is, with sacrificing the spirit to the letter by overlooking graver cruelties while denouncing minor ones—we should have been fully prepared to meet so serious an accusation. But as they have not done this, but have merely twitted us with not attempting everything at once, and with allowing the subordinate evil to wait until the central evil has been grappled with, we cheerfully admit the impeachment—coming as it does (such is the humour of the situation) from those who are themselves desirous of perpetuating *both* kinds of suffering, the greater and the smaller alike! We beg to assure them that we would much rather be inconsistently humane than consistently cruel.

THE DEGRADATION OF THE BUTCHER

But this question of butchery is not merely one of kindness or unkindness to animals, for by the very facts of the case it is a *human* question of no slight importance, affecting as it does the social and moral welfare of those more immediately concerned in it. Of all recognised occupations by which in civilised countries a livelihood is sought and obtained, the work which is looked upon with the greatest loathing (next to the hangman's) is that of the butcher—as witness the opprobrious sense which the word "butcher" has acquired. Owing to the instinctive horror of bloodshed, which is characteristic of all normal civilised beings, the trade of doing to death countless numbers of inoffensive and highly-organised creatures amid scenes of indescribable filth and ferocity is delegated—in the large towns, at any rate—to a pariah class of "slaughtermen," who are thus themselves made the victims of a grievous social wrong. "I'm only doing your dirty work. It's such as *you* makes such as *us*," is said to have been the remark of a Whitechapel butcher to a flesh-eating gentleman who remonstrated with him for his brutality; and the remark was a perfectly just one. To demand a product which can only be procured at the cost of the intense suffering of the animal and the deep degradation of the butcher, and by a process which not one flesh-eater in a hundred would himself under any circumstances perform or even witness, is conduct as callous, selfish, and unsocial as could well be imagined.

For butchery, as Sir Benjamin Richardson used to point out, is essentially a "dangerous trade." It not only deadens and destroys the moral sympathies, but it has the physical effect of straining the nerves and weakening the heart of the slaughterman, and thus naturally induces a tendency to have recourse to drink. How often, too, in reading of some murderous crime, has one seen it stated that the criminal was a butcher; as, for instance, in the Austrian "ripper" case, when, as the papers stated, a woman of the "unfortunate" class was killed by a young butcher of herculean frame, by whom it is supposed a previous victim had also been slaughtered. To have accustomed one's self to a total disregard for the pleading terror of sensitive animals and to a murderous use of the knife is a terrible power for society to put into the hands of its lowest and least responsible members.

The blame must ultimately fall on society itself, and not on the individual slaughterman. No one had a better knowledge of this subject than the late Mr. H. F. Lester, and this is his opinion:

> "We must take into consideration the fact that the ranks of slaughtermen are habitually made up from persons in whom one could hardly expect to find the sentiment of pity strongly developed; yet, even among these, there is a certain air of dissatisfaction with the work they are compelled to do, and a mixture of insolence and shamefacedness, of swagger and evident dislike of inspection, which makes one think they know their trade is a nasty one, only bearable from lack of other employment and from the good wages earned. But there are plenty of men engaged in this work of killing animals for food who are much too good for the business. These will tell you openly that they dislike the job, but 'people will have meat,' and if they were to give it up, someone else would step into the work."[18]

Again, subordinate to the actual butchery, there are certain disgusting, if not dangerous, occupations, such as that of the women who work in or near the cattle markets at the malodorous task of "preparing animal entrails for commercial uses," of which process the following account has been given:[19] "The women's share in the ugly business begins when the greasy, slimy intestinal skins come to them for the scraping off of all fat and substance still attaching to them. They are washed, twisted up, dressed with salt, and are ready for the sausage-makers, on whose behalf they have been thus prepared." The journalistic comment is, that "in an ideal world men would not permit women to do work from which every instinct of refinement and even decency shrinks," but that all is over-ruled by "the demands of present-day cheapness." This, as things go, is undeniable; but it would be well that conscientious flesh-eaters should at least realise what their diet imposes on other people.

That, however, is just what they are mostly determined *not* to realise, doubtless from a subconscious apprehension that, if once they begin to look into this unsavoury subject, they may be pushed to the verge of certain awkward conclusions. Nothing is more significant than the extreme unwillingness of philanthropists and members of ethical societies, who debate almost every problem under the sun, to give serious attention to the question of butchery—a reluctance which may be taken as one of the strongest possible tributes to the pertinence of vegetarianism. This is said to be especially true of the philanthropists of Chicago—that great centre of the killing trade. "No one who goes to Chicago," says an eye-witness, "should fail to see the shambles. They are the most wicked things in creation. They are sickening beyond description. The men in them are more brutes than the animals they slaughter. Missions and institutes have been built in the respectable parts of the city from the profits, and the employees of the shambles have been left to go straight down to the devil.... It is the duty of everyone interested in social questions, of everyone whose demands necessitate this kind of labour, to wade through this filth to see these poor wretches at work."[20]

And so they go their ways, the philanthropist to build "homes," the ethical folk to talk learnedly, and the social reformer to concoct schemes for the amelioration of the human race. Yet, meantime, these very persons are themselves perpetuating, by their mode of living, the evil conditions which they profess to be anxious to remove, and condemning the pariah slaughterman to a life of sheer bestiality. "The meat-eater," says Mr. Lester, "accepts the results of this man's demoralisation of character. Pious and professed Christians are content to allow the deep degradation of the nature of a whole class of men, set apart to do the nation's dirty work of slaughtering, without an apparent thought of the baseness of their conduct."

Here, as I said at the outset, is a distinctively *human* question, and one which cannot be evaded, even by those slippery reasoners who would shuffle out of the duty of humaneness to animals by pretending (in the face of evolutionary science) that there is no bond of consanguinity between the animals and mankind. By no possible sophistry can "educated" people be justified in placing this heavy burden of butchery on the hands of their social "inferiors." The vivisector and the sportsman have at least the courage to do their own devilries; and the work even of the hardened agents of "murderous millinery" and the fur-trade is diversified to some extent by travel and adventure. But the slaughterman's task is one of unrelieved, unmitigated brutality, involving the constant and systematic doing of deeds that are inhuman in themselves, degrading to the rough men who do them, and trebly disgraceful to the polite ladies and gentlemen at whose behest they are done.

THE ÆSTHETIC ARGUMENT

Closely connected with the humane argument is the æsthetic argument, the two being, in fact, twin branches of the same stem. For "humane," as the Latin shows, has the double meaning of "gentle" and "refined"; so that "humanity," in the original conception of the term, implies not only a moral regard for the rights of our fellow-beings, but also an æsthetic appreciation of what is beautiful and pure. Culture and good-breeding, together with justice and compassion, are the characteristics of humane man; and the fact that this twofold sense of the word has been well-nigh forgotten in the education of the modern "gentleman" may serve to explain why there is often such a grievous lack of gentleness in persons who claim to be refined. Our *literæ humaniores* are a mere academic course of book-learning, the *humane* element being altogether left out of account; and to such bathos has this divorce of gentleness and refinement carried us that, in some quarters, a "professor of humanity" is—a teacher of Latin grammar.

We are prepared, then, to find that the æsthetic or artistic faculty of the present day is deplorably narrow in its scope, and is so ignorant of the true relationship of humanity and art that it actually prides itself on omitting from its ken all humane considerations, while it diligently searches for the beautiful and the picturesque, as if beauty were a thing detached from the realities of every-day life! The bare idea that there is an æsthetic side to the diet question, beyond the mere delicacies of cookery and embellishments of the dining-table, would be scouted as ridiculous by ninety-nine out of a hundred of our artists or literary men; for the very force of habit which has made them so quick to resent the least technical flaw in their special departments of work, has left them blindly indifferent to the hideous and revolting aspects of flesh-eating. To these æsthetes, so-called, the sight of an ugly house, for example, is a sore trouble and grievance, but the slaughter-house, with all its gruesome doings, is a matter of supreme unconcern—nay, rather a thing to be indirectly patronised and defended. I have known a case where an æsthetic lady, of great personal culture, and the centre of a polished circle, stained the floor of her charming suburban villa with bullock's blood brought from the shambles in a bucket.

Yet the æsthete does not usually vindicate his carnivorous diet and its appurtenances with the old unhesitating heartiness of the barbarian; he is somewhat ashamed of himself—unconsciously, perhaps—in these latter days, even as the cannibal is ashamed when the discussion turns upon "long pig." Like all the apologists of flesh-eating, in their respective spheres, he is shifty and evasive in his defences, and is not too proud, in his moment of extremity, to have recourse to the "consistency trick," and to try to trip up his vegetarian persecutor with the retort of "You're another." From which signs of grace it may be surmised that the æsthete, in spite of his brave exterior, is not quite at ease in his dietetic philosophy, and that the products of butchery are, in a very real sense, the "skeleton in the cupboard" (the larder cupboard) of literature and art.

ÆSTHETE: Pray, why do you address yourself to *me* in that significant manner?

VEGETARIAN: Because I understand that you cultivate the artistic sense. You love to have beautiful things about you, do you not? So you must needs wish to be a vegetarian.

ÆSTHETE: I love beautiful things, certainly. Art is my vocation. But what has vegetarianism to do with it?

VEGETARIAN: Have the arrangements of the dinner-table nothing to do with it—the cloth, the silver, the glasses, the dessert, the flowers?

ÆSTHETE: A great deal, obviously. There is much art in dining well.

VEGETARIAN: Yet the meats that are served at the table have nothing to do with it! Is not that rather contradictory?

ÆSTHETE: I did not say that. The cookery is an essential point, of course.

VEGETARIAN: But what of the meat—the thing cooked? What *is* it? What *was* it? And how did it come to be on your plate?

ÆSTHETE: I never think of such questions. So long as it is nice, I am content. It must satisfy my taste, that is all.

VEGETARIAN: But are you sure that it *does* satisfy your taste in the same way that other things do? I think not, for you have never put it to the trial. In no other branch of art do you take things wholly on trust, but you try them by the standard of an independent and educated intelligence. In diet, and in diet only, you "shut your eyes and open your mouth," as the children say, and never distinguish between a real innate liking and the liking that is merely traditional.

ÆSTHETE: *De gustibus non est disputandum.*

VEGETARIAN: About genuine tastes, I admit, disputation is idle. But the proverb is not true of the sham tastes to which I refer. There is a great deal to be discussed about *them*.

ÆSTHETE: But I assure you my liking for a ham-sandwich is a genuine taste.

VEGETARIAN: With full knowledge of the pig-sty and the pig-sticker. Do not the antecedents of your ham-sandwich cause you a feeling of disgust?

ÆSTHETE: Oh, well, if you persist in thinking about it, *all* feeding causes disgust. Don't you think there is something gross in the whole process of ingestion?

VEGETARIAN: Then why not gorge on carrion at once? The moment you adopt the "in for a penny, in for a pound" attitude, you sacrifice the whole art of living.

ÆSTHETE: But what of the processes on which vegetarianism itself depends? You talk of the filth of the slaughter-house; but how about the filth of market gardening? To watch the soil being manured, if we let our thoughts dwell upon it, is enough to spoil all appetite for the produce of the garden. The more delicious the asparagus or the strawberries, the more we ought to loathe them.

VEGETARIAN: There I disagree with you entirely. There is nothing in the least disgusting, to me, at any rate (and I speak from personal experience), in the manuring of the soil or in any agricultural process—on the contrary, there is much that is wholesome and cheering in this chemistry of nature. The healthy mind takes a delight in gardening, just as it regards slaughtering with abhorrence. If you want to see the contrast between the effects of the two professions on those who practise them, compare the face of the typical slaughterman with that of the typical gardener. It is as remarkable as the contrast between a butcher's and a fruiterer's shop.

ÆSTHETE: Well, it is no use talking about it; our views of life are different. You are a social reformer and agitator, and agitation is fatal to the tranquility of art. I am an artist, and do not care a straw for social reform. My creed is expressed in Keats's couplet:

Beauty is truth, truth beauty—that is all
Ye know on earth, and all ye need to know.

VEGETARIAN: Yes, but it is possible that Keats's meaning is somewhat deeper than you imagine. It is not your creed that I quarrel with, but your own misunderstanding and misuse of it. That the oneness of truth and beauty is knowledge sufficient, I admit; but my complaint is that you do *not* really know it, and therefore I regard your æstheticism—the æstheticism that makes clean the outside of the cup and the platter, and the outside only—as mere vandalism in masquerade.

Nor is even the outside of the æsthetic platter free from offence, for there is nothing more hideous to the eye (not to mention the mind) than the "scorched corpses," as Bernard Shaw calls them, that are displayed on polite dinner-tables when the dish-covers are removed. "Among the customs at table that deserve to be abolished," wrote Leigh Hunt, "is that of serving up dishes that retain a look of life in death—codfish with their staring eyes, hares with their hollow countenances, etc. It is in bad taste, an incongruity, an anomaly; to say nothing of its effect on morbid imaginations." Perhaps, however, the most morbid imagination, or lack of imagination, is that of the persons who are *not* disgusted by these ugly sights.

Art and humanity, then, are but two branches of the same stock: the true humanist and the true artist are own brethren. To the artistic temperament, in particular, vegetarianism has the surest right of appeal; for the æstheticism which can prate of truth and beauty, while it battens like a ghoul on bloodshed and suffering, has abnegated its own principles, and has ceased to be artistic. How would it be possible for the scenes that are hourly enacted in slaughter-houses to be tolerated for a moment in a community which had any real artistic consciousness? Yet what "æsthetic" protest, except from vegetarians, is ever raised against them? Take, for example, the following extract from some notes descriptive of the Chicago meat factories:

> "Slithered over bloody floor. Nearly broke neck in gore of old porker. Saw few hundred men slicing pigs, making hams, sausages, and pork chops. Whole sight not edifying; indeed, rather beastly. Next went to cattle-killing house. Cattle driven along gangway and banged over head with iron hammer. Fell stunned; then swung up by legs, and man cuts throats. Small army of men with buckets catching blood; it gushed over them in torrents—a bit sickening. Next to sheep slaughter-house. More throat-cutting—ten thousand sheep killed a day—more blood. Place reeks with blood; walls and floor splashed with it; air thick, warm, offensive. 'Yes,' said guide, 'Armour's biggest slaughter-house in the world. There's no waste; we utilise everything—everything except the squeak of the pigs. We can't can that.' Went and drank brandy."[21]

It is much to be regretted that it is not found possible, in this enterprising establishment, to "can" the squeak, as well as the flesh, of the pig; for such a phonographic effect might suggest certain novel thoughts to the refined ladies and gentlemen who contentedly regale themselves on ham-sandwiches at polite supper-tables. For imagine what the result would be, in studio and boudoir, dining-room and drawing-room, if the death-cries of the slaughter-house could be but once uncanned and brought to hearing. "The groans and screams of this poor persecuted race," as De Quincey said of cats, "if gathered into some great echoing hall of horrors, would melt the heart of the stoniest." But far vaster and more impressive would be the world-wide hall of horrors which should contain the bitter cry of the victims of the butcher. Would that it were possible thus to compel the æsthetic flesh-eater to "face the music" of his misdeeds!

And, remember, it is not only at the big slaughtering centres that these ugly trades are carried on, nor are they there, perhaps, at their ugliest; but every town and every village has its private torture-dens where the same carnage is performed the year round on a smaller scale and in a clumsier manner, and everywhere the butcher's shop presents the same ghastly spectacle of quartered carcases hanging a-row, and gloated over by "shopping" women. One would think it incredible that any lover of the beautiful could doubt that the national sense of beauty must be seriously impaired by these disgusting and degrading sights. But enough of the subject! Were we to dwell too long on it, we should be tempted to exclaim, as was said of another kind of iniquity, "While these things are being done, beauty stands veiled, and music is a screeching lie."

THE HYGIENIC ARGUMENT

The humane and the æsthetic aspects of vegetarianism are constantly described by the advocates of flesh-eating as "sentimental," and if it be sentimental to have regard for the sufferings of animals and the beauty of our own surroundings, the charge will be gladly admitted; but there is also, independent of all considerations of humanity, a distinctly hygienic movement towards the disuse of flesh food, on the ground that such diet is not only barbarous but unwholesome. It is held that flesh food is in itself a stimulant, and that incidentally it is very liable to transmit disease, while vegetarianism, on the contrary, is a simple, natural, less inflammatory diet, which from the earliest times has been known and practised by a few wise persons as containing the secret of health. In Germany, especially, the system of "natural living" has attracted much attention, and the propaganda of food reform is there mainly on those lines; in England less so, but here, too, there are a number of vegetarians who are hygienists first and humanitarians afterwards, and all humanitarians are to some extent hygienists, so that it is ridiculous, in any serious criticism of vegetarianism, to leave out of sight, as some of our opponents do, this essential part of the system.

There is, in fact, a considerable scientific literature on the subject, a train of thought and experience handed down from Cornaro and Gassendi, through their successors Cheyne, Hartley, Lambe, Abernethy, and others, to such modern authorities as Sir Benjamin Richardson and Dr. Alexander Haig; yet so little known is this testimony that it might be imagined, from the nervous apprehension with which the abandonment of flesh flood is regarded, that vegetarianism were some new and hazardous experiment, whereon he who enters carries his life in his hands. This ignorance of the long-standing claims of vegetarianism to a scientific basis is the result of the indifference and prejudice that have always made dietetics the most unpopular of studies, those who are in health not caring to give more than a passing thought to the hygienic quality of their food, while those who are sick are naturally suspicious of change or over-ruled by medical advisers.

Yet the moment impartial inquiry is made into the comparative benefits and perils of the two modes of living, certain undeniable facts begin to appear, of which the first and most obvious, though not the most important, perhaps, are the *incidental* dangers of flesh-eating. Many, indeed, and unsuspected by the ordinary man who takes a "good meat dinner," are the ills that flesh is heir to, especially in the diet of the poor; for, as Professor F. W. Newman pointed out, "where the population is dense, the poorer classes, if they eat flesh-meat at all, are sure to get a sensible portion of their supply in an unwholesome state." This assertion is no mere piece of vegetarian polemics; it rests on the authority of more than one Royal Commission, the latest of which has insisted, in the Tuberculosis Report of 1898, that "so long as private slaughter-houses are permitted to exist, so long must inspection be carried out under conditions incompatible with efficiency." There is, in fact, no genuine inspection of the meat killed in private slaughter-houses, nor is the case (at present) much better in public ones, and it is notorious that a large amount of tuberculous flesh, examined and rejected under their more careful scrutiny by the Jews, is thought good enough to be sold for the use of the "Gentiles." It would be easy to quote official figures to show the prevalence of the mischief, but it is not necessary here to do so, because the facts are not denied.[22] The cause of the disease thus prevalent among cattle must be sought partly in the excessive demand for flesh food, and the consequent high price of meat, which is a great temptation to graziers to breed from immature stock; partly, too, in the unhealthy system of stall-feeding and cramming, and last, but not least, in the rough treatment to which animals are exposed during their transit by sea and rail—an evil which is recognised by butchers no less than by humanitarians.

Moreover, in addition to the dangers which flesh-eaters incur of diseases contagious and parasitic, there is the risk of eating decomposed meat under the title of "table delicacies." Here, as one instance out of many, is an extract from a London daily paper.

> Some exemplary fines were inflicted when summonses connected with the seizure of 13 tons of rotten pigs' livers came on for hearing. A company promoter, trading as manufacturer of table delicacies, was fined £100, including costs, for the possession of forty-four barrels of the livers, which were deposited for the purpose of being converted into human food in the shape of meat-extracts, soups, and other table delicacies. The magistrate characterised the condemned goods as "absolute filth."

The bearing of such facts on the public health is obvious. "The shocking revelations," it has been said, "as to the potted meat trade of London, clearly give us the key-note to the terrible weekly statistics of fevers and other diseases in the poorer districts of London and big towns generally. Putrid sheep's hearts—putrid meat of unknown origin—anything from horse to pug dog—slimy livers, reeking lights that would poison even a Fleet Street cat, and moribund hams from diseased pigs are the foundation of our table delicacies. Ugh! it is enough to make a man forswear anything 'potted' for ever."[23]

But, though these and similar facts are indisputable, and though so great an authority as Sir B. W. Richardson has stated that, "in respect to the propagation of disease, it seems just to declare that the danger is much less and much more easily preventable on the vegetarian than on the animal diet," the flesh-eaters, strong or weak as they may happen to be, even to the sickliest valetudinarian that ever sipped his Liebig, are much more afraid of being infected with vegetarian principles than with the poisons of the murdered ox, and would venture on every drug in the Pharmacopœia rather than on a pure and simple diet. Yet more than a hundred and fifty years ago so eminent a physician as Dr. George Cheyne, then in a hale old age, had written as follows:

> "My regimen at present is milk, with tea, coffee, bread-and-butter, mild cheese, salads, fruits and seeds of all kinds, with tender roots (as potatoes, turnips, carrots), and, in short, everything that has not life, dressed or not, as I like, in which there is as much or a greater variety than in animal foods, so that the stomach need never be cloyed. I drink no wine nor any fermented liquors, and am rarely dry, most of my food being liquid, moist, or juicy. Only after dinner I drink either coffee or green tea, but seldom both in the same day, and sometimes a glass of soft small cider. The thinner my diet, the easier, more cheerful and lightsome I find myself; my sleep is also the sounder, though perhaps somewhat shorter than formerly under my full animal diet; but, then, I am more alive than ever I was."[24]

The close connection of vegetarianism with temperance, simplicity, and general hardihood has been discovered by many thousands of persons since Dr. Cheyne recorded it, and has had its latest illustration in the doings of vegetarian athletes, whose remarkable achievements in cycling matches and long-distance walks have shown once more that flesh-eating is not by any means a necessary condition of physical prowess. It cannot be mere accident that vegetarians are almost invariably abstainers from alcohol and tobacco, that, man for man, they eat more sparingly, dress more lightly, live more naturally, and work harder than flesh-eaters, and are far less subject to illnesses and ailments. It is notorious that in quite a number of diseases, especially those of the gouty class, a vegetarian diet is prescribed by medical men, who use for *cure* what they scorn to use for *prevention*. In the works of Dr. Alexander Haig,[25] the most distinguished recent exponent of reformed diet, a close study has been made of the comparative wholesomeness and unwholesomeness of vegetable and animal foods, and to these writings, together with those of the other authorities above-mentioned, I would refer any of my readers who may be under the idea that vegetarianism has no medical support. The doctors, of course, or those of them who study the history of their own profession, are well aware of the hollowness of this common superstition, but they still continue to let an ignorant public fondly hug the belief that vegetarianism is a mere "fad," a mushroom growth born of the follies and sentimentalities of a decadent and hypercivilised age.

It is impossible in the limit of these pages, which are concerned with the logical, not the medical view of vegetarianism, to discuss with any fulness the argument based on hygiene; but it may be stated as a matter, not of opinion, but of knowledge, that quite apart from all humane bias, there is a strong case for the reformed regimen on the ground of its healthfulness alone, and that a scientific statement of this case may be found, by those who care to become acquainted with the facts, in the published writings of a small, but not inconsiderable succession of medical authorities. Humanity and hygiene are the twin deities of food reform, and their paths, though separate for the time, converge eventually to the same vegetarian goal.

DIGESTION

We have seen that the scientific apologists of flesh-eating do not seriously rely on the old bogey of "structural evidence," though they have certainly not been over-anxious to dissociate their cause from whatever support has accrued to it through this too common misunderstanding. The same is true of that other widespread superstition, that meat alone "gives strength"—*i.e.*, that vegetarian diet, as compared with a flesh diet, is deficient in flesh-forming constituents—an error which the medical faculty, as a whole, has secretly fostered and encouraged, though in face of the existence of the elephant and rhinoceros and other mighty herbivora, its responsible spokesmen have, of course, not committed themselves to any such absurdity. Except for the fact that thousands of ignorant persons are still under the delusion that no adequate nourishment is to be found in the vegetable kingdom, it would not be necessary to point out that, by the admission of all authorities, the albuminoids, carbohydrates, oils, salts, and other chemical food-properties, exist in vegetable no less than in animal substances, and therefore that a vegetarian diet, even without the use of eggs and milk, has access to all the needed elements.

The professional, as distinct from the popular, objections to vegetarianism, are based nowadays on quite other arguments, as may be seen from the suggestive admissions and assertions made in the following passage from the *British Medical Journal*:

> "Man is undoubtedly in his anatomy most nearly allied to the higher apes, and these animals, though they show obvious tendencies to be omnivorous, are yet, in the main, eaters of nuts and fruits. But man is not a higher ape, and in the process of development to his present high status he has become omnivorous. It is true that he can obtain from vegetables the nutriment necessary for his maintenance in health, but he has learnt that *he can obtain what he wants at less cost of energy from a mixed diet*, and he is not likely to unlearn this lesson."[26]

In the words that I have italicised we have the latest shibboleth of carnivorous "science" in its changing treatment of the food question. Vegetarianism is not "impossible" (as we used to be told it was)! Oh, no! life, and even healthy life, can really be maintained on a diet of vegetables (how many thousands of doctors have asserted the contrary!). But the inferior *digestibility* of vegetable food—that is the trouble! The poor vegetarians must put their digestive organs to so great a strain, and must eat so large a bulk of food in order to get the requisite nourishment. Why, then, says the chemist, should they thus over-tax their systems, when they could digest a few slices from a dead body at so much less cost of energy?

Now, if the chemist were a man of action, and not merely a man of study, the practical aspects of this question might at the outset give him pause. Had he known vegetarians, lived among vegetarians, and talked with vegetarians, instead of regarding them theoretically, he would be aware that the average vegetarian eats decidedly *less* in bulk than the average flesh-eater, and is seldom or never troubled with the indigestion that the flesh-eater dreads. So far from being compelled to consume a greater bulk of food, it is the general experience of those who have adopted vegetarianism that they eat much less under the new system than they did under the old, and it is a frequent marvel to them, when they dine with their former messmates, to see the huge amounts that they devour.

There is the further consideration, entirely overlooked in the argument of the *British Medical Journal*, that "vegetarianism," in the current sense of the word, is not a diet of vegetables only, but includes the use of eggs, butter, cheese, and milk. For all which reasons the talk about "less cost of energy" seems to have little practical bearing on the subject under discussion, and it may be suspected that the chemical chimera is quite as fabulous as the phantom difficulties that have preceded it.

CHEMIST: Now listen! I am a chemist, and I have no time to think or talk of anything sentimental. To all your views about vegetarian diet I have but one answer—"Hofmann's experiments."

VEGETARIAN: So Hofmann's figures have settled this diet problem for all time?

CHEMIST: Undoubtedly. For they prove that the human stomach can assimilate a greater percentage of animal than of vegetable substances; in other words, that it requires a greater exercise of digestive power to get an equal amount of nourishment from vegetables. What have you to say to that?

VEGETARIAN: Obviously this—that it is quite devoid of value unless we know *who* were the persons experimented on. No statistics of the comparative digestibility of foods can be of practical use unless the habits and conditions of those who digest the foods are also noted. Custom and the personal element are all-important factors in the result. Many vegetable foods, nuts for example, are readily digested by vegetarians accustomed to their use, though almost universally found indigestible by flesh-eaters.

CHEMIST: I cannot follow you into that. Let us keep clear of all such sentiment, if you please, and bear in mind the great precept which Dr. Andrew Wilson, in his application of Hofmann's figures, has laid down for our guidance, that "animal matter, being likest to our own composition, is most easily and readily converted into ourselves."

VEGETARIAN: With all due deference to the Andrew Wilson formula, may I ask what matter *is* likest to our own?

CHEMIST: Why, *animal* matter, of course.

VEGETARIAN: Yes, but *what* animal matter?

CHEMIST: Oh, we don't go into that.

VEGETARIAN: But I do; and I beg you to observe that the "matter likest to our own composition" is *human* flesh, so that according to the Andrew Wilson formula, we all ought to be cannibals, because for human beings human flesh must be the most digestible of foods.

CHEMIST: Very likely it is so, though I do not approve of cannibalism.

VEGETARIAN: Then allow me to read you a sentence from C. F. Gordon Cumming's book, "At Home in Fiji." "At every cannibal feast there was served a certain vegetable, also commonly used by the cannibal Maoris of New Zealand, which was considered as essential an adjunct as mint-sauce is to lamb or sage to goose. Its use, however, was prudential, as human flesh *was found to be highly indigestible*, and this herb acted as a corrective." Now I ask you if that does not logically dispose of the Andrew Wilson formula?

CHEMIST: Nonsense, sir! I will not discuss cannibalism. You fail to see that some things, though logical enough, may not be expedient.

VEGETARIAN: I am delighted to hear you say that. I beg you to remember it when you next talk of "Hofmann's experiments." It is possible that flesh-eating, like cannibalism, is "not expedient," when it is regarded from a wider standpoint than that of the chemical doctrinaire.

Nothing, indeed, could be more *un*scientific than the attitude taken on this question by "scientists" of the Andrew Wilson type. For, in the first place, as pointed out above, it is impossible to arrive at any scientific conclusion as to the comparative digestibility of vegetable and animal foods unless the conditions are equal—that is, unless the persons experimented on are equally accustomed to the food-stuffs they are invited to digest; and, secondly, there is the question of the quality of the foods supplied, for as Dr. Oldfield has remarked, "it is quite as unfair to judge of the digestibility of the proteid of the vegetable kingdom from one example of the legumens as it would be to class all forms of flesh as indigestible because veal or lobster happens to be so." Against the academic testimony of the Hofmann school of specialists we may confidently set that of so distinguished a practical chemist as Sir B. W. Richardson, who, by his personal knowledge of vegetarians and vegetarianism, was peculiarly qualified to judge. "From experimental observations which I have made, I am of opinion that the vegetable flesh-forming substances may be as easily digested, when they are presented to the stomach in proper form, as are the animal substances of like feeding quality."[27]

The true function of the chemist in his general relation to the diet question is to help the coming dietary by transferring to the vegetarian system some of the scientific attention that has hitherto been solely devoted to flesh meats. "Men of practical science," says Sir B. W. Richardson, "ought to be at work assisting with their skill in bringing about that mighty reformation. We now know to a nicety the relation of the various parts of food needed for the construction of the living body, and there should be no difficulty, except the labour of research, in so modifying food from its prime source as to make it applicable to every necessity without the assistance of any intermediate animal at all." Why should not the chemist, instead of maintaining, like Mrs. Partington, a pettifogging and quite futile opposition to the flowing tide, put himself in the current of progress, and try to turn his special knowledge to the furtherance of a noble end?

CONDITIONS OF CLIMATE

To try to "change the venue" is sometimes the policy of defendants in an action at law, and a similar device is adopted by those who would stave off the hearing of the vegetarian case. "The tropics" are the convenient limbo to which this uncongenial subject is most frequently consigned; and it is with a proud sense of humour and self-assurance that the British Islander, who objects to alien immigration and all foreign frivolities, warns the vegetarian heresy to keep clear of his inhospitable clime. Such diet may be all very well, he thinks, for passive Hindoos, but not for the hard-working inhabitants of this temperate zone.

BRITISH ISLANDER: Vegetarianism? No thank you; not *here*! All very nice in Africa and India, I dare say, where you can sit all day under a palm-tree and eat dates.

VEGETARIAN: But I have not observed that when you visit Africa or India you practise vegetarianism. On the contrary, you take your flesh-pots with you everywhere—even to the very places where you admit you don't need them, and where, as in India, they give the greatest offence to the inhabitants.

BRITISH ISLANDER: Oh, well, it's no affair of theirs, is it, if I take my roast beef?

VEGETARIAN: Yet you think it your affair to interfere with the cannibals when they take their roast man. And have you observed that it is in the tropical zone, not the temperate zone, that cannibalism is most rife?

BRITISH ISLANDER: Why do you remind me of that?

VEGETARIAN: To show you that all this talk about vegetarianism being "a matter of climate" is pure humbug. The use of flesh is a vicious habit everywhere, and nowhere a necessity, except where other food is not procurable.

BRITISH ISLANDER: But do we not need more oil and fat in northern climates?

VEGETARIAN: Undoubtedly; but these can be readily obtained without recourse to flesh.

BRITISH ISLANDER: Then how do you account for the fact that northern races have been, to so great an extent, carnivorous?

VEGETARIAN: Perhaps because in primitive times hunting and pasturage were less toilsome than agriculture. But I am not called on to "account" for such a fact. Their past addiction to flesh food no more proves the present utility of flesh-eating than their gross drinking habits prove the utility of alcohol.

BRITISH ISLANDER: Can you quote any scientific authority for your contention?

VEGETARIAN: There is one which is all the more valuable because it is an admission made by an opponent. Sir William Lawrence wrote: "That men can be perfectly nourished, and that their physical and intellectual capabilities can be fully developed in any climate by a diet purely vegetable, has been proved by such abundant experience that it will not be necessary to adduce any formal arguments on the subject."[28] "In any climate," mark! And a diet "purely vegetable"; whereas all *you* are asked to do is to forego the actual flesh foods, and not the animal products. But come now! Ask me the great question!

BRITISH ISLANDER: What is that? There is only one other I had in mind. What would become of the Esquimaux?

VEGETARIAN: Of course! I have always been profoundly touched by the disinterested concern of the Englishman (when vegetarianism looms ahead) for the future of that Arctic people. Well, perhaps the question of what ice-bound savages might do, or might not do, need scarcely delay the decision of civilised mankind. For that matter, what would become of the polar bears? If you cannot dissociate your habits from those of the Esquimaux, why don't you eat blubber? At least they have a better reason for eating blubber than some people have for eating beef—they can get nothing else.

The dishonesty of the excuse that vegetarianism "may be all very well in the tropics" is shown by the fact that Englishmen, when living in the tropics, make precisely the contrary statement. "You would be surprised," writes Mr. B. K. Adams, from Ceylon, "if you knew how much prejudice and opposition there is here. The most amusing part is that nearly everyone says, it is all very well being a vegetarian in England, in a cool climate like that, but out here in this hot, depressing, and enervating climate, you must have meat, and some add alcoholic stimulant."[29]

Twenty years ago, just the same "climatic" argument used to be put forward by the opponents of the temperance movement; it was impossible *here* to abstain from alcoholic drink, whatever it might be elsewhere. We do not often meet with that argument now; on the contrary, it is generally admitted that a disuse of alcohol brings with it an increased power of hardihood and endurance. As in drink, so in food. Those who fly to stimulants obtain a temporary sense of comfort at the cost of permanent vigour.

But granting that it is possible to support life on vegetarian diet in northern climates, is it also possible, asks the conscientious doubter, to live at one's highest energy under such conditions? Look at the carnivorous Mr. Dash's career, it is said, as compared with that of the vegetarian Mr. So-and-So! Was not the greater public activity of the former attributable to his mixed diet? To which it may be replied that any such personal comparison is necessarily useless, from lack of sufficient data as to the relative powers and opportunities of the persons compared. It is obvious that a man whose convictions are unpopular will have far less opportunity of carrying his principles into action than one who is the mouthpiece of widely current opinions, to the propagation of which he devotes, perhaps, an equal amount of ability. For this reason it is absurd to suggest that vegetarians, or any other class of unpopular reformers, are living on a less active plane because their activities are not of the kind that commend themselves to the man in the street—or to that equally fallible person, the man in the study.

The whole notion that vegetarians are less able than flesh-eaters to endure a severe climate is a delusion; it is not only untrue, but the contrary of the truth. "No one surely suggests," says Dr. Oldfield, "that the English climate is too cold for a vegetarian dietary, when there is the experience of the stalwart, hardy Scotch peasantry, in a climate far more rigorous, developing brain and muscle superior

54

to the average Englishman, and this upon a dietary which for generations has been so largely vegetarian that no one would dream of saying that the small amount of flesh eaten by them could have had anything to do with the matter."[30]

Anyone who is intimately acquainted with the vegetarian movement in this country will bear me out when I say that the average vegetarian is much less susceptible than the average flesh-eater to extremes of cold and heat, and can get through an English winter in comparative comfort, without any of the "wrapping up" to which the mixed dietists are reduced. It is amusing, indeed, after being asked that common question, "Don't you feel the cold very much, as you eat no meat?" to observe one's questioner attired perhaps to face a moderate London winter like a German student for a duel—a moving mass of scarves and furs and overcoats, stoked up internally with plates of beef and cups of bovril, and shivering withal. "Poor fellow!" one thinks, "it looks as if *you* were the person whose diet might be all very well for those who live in the tropics, but not for the hard-working inhabitants of this northern clime."

FLESH MEAT AND MORALS

"Man is what he eats," says the materialist in the German proverb. The body is built up of the food-stuffs which it assimilates, and it is reasonable to suppose that diet has thus a determining influence on character. If this be true, the reflection is not a pleasant one for the flesh-eater. "Animal food," it has been said, "containing as it does highly-wrought organic forces, may liberate within our system powers which we may find it difficult or even impossible to dominate— lethargic monsters, foul harpies, and sad-visaged lemurs—which may insist on having their own way, building up an animal body not truly human."[31]

But here the idealist steps in with a different theory. Man is not what he eats, but what he thinks and feels; it is not *what* we eat, but *how* we eat, that most vitally affects us. This is well expressed in one of Thoreau's daring paradoxes: "There is a certain class of unbelievers who sometimes ask me such questions as if I think I can live on vegetable food alone; and to strike at the root of the matter at once— for the root is faith—I am accustomed to answer such, that I can live on board-nails. If they cannot understand that, they cannot understand much that I have to say."

There is, however, no real antagonism between these two theories, for both may be to a great extent true, though neither wholly so. If mind affects matter, matter also affects mind; if spirit acts on food, food in its turn reacts on spirit. The one truth that stands out clearly from a consideration of this subject, and from the witness of common experience, is that a gross animal diet is inimical to the finer instincts, and that, as Thoreau says, "every man who has ever been earnest to preserve his higher or more poetic faculties in the best condition, has been particularly inclined to abstain from animal food."[32] Plain living and high thinking are indissolubly connected. Vegetarianism, as I have already shown, is not asceticism, but if it offer the moral advantages of asceticism without the drawbacks, is not that in its favour?

But there is a tendency among certain "psychical" authorities of the present day to eschew the vegetarian doctrine as itself "materialistic," and as attributing too much importance to the mere bodily functions of eating and digesting. "What does it matter about our diet," they say, "whether it be animal or vegetable, flesh or fruit, so long as the spirit in which we seek it be a fit and proper one? The question of food is one for doctors to decide; 'tis they who are concerned with the body, while we are concerned with the soul." I wish to show that this reasoning is nothing but a piece of charlatanry, and rests upon a perversion of the philosophy that it claims to represent.

For though it is true, in a sense, that spirit can sanctify diet, it is not true that a general sanction is thereby given to any diet whatsoever, no matter what cruelties may be caused by it, or who it be that causes them. We may grant that so long as no scruple has arisen concerning the morality of flesh-eating, or any other barbarous usage, such practices may be carried on in innocence and good faith, and therefore without personal demoralisation to those who indulge in them. But from the moment when discussion begins, and an unconscious act becomes a conscious or semi-conscious one, the case is wholly different, and it is then impossible to plead that "it does not matter" about one's food. On the contrary, it is a matter of vital import if injustice be deliberately practised. To use flesh food unwittingly, by savage instinct, as the carnivora do, or, like barbarous mankind, in the ignorance of age-long habit, is one thing; but it is quite another thing for a rational person to make a sophistical defence of such habits when their iniquity has been displayed, and *then* to claim that he is absolved from guilt by the spirit in which he acted. The spirit that absolves is one of unquestioning faith, not of far-fetched sophistry. The wolf devours the lamb, and is no worse a wolf for it; but if he seek, as in the fable, to give quibbling excuses for his wolfishness, he becomes a byword for hypocrisy.

PSYCHIC PHILOSOPHER: Why all this fuss about vegetarianism and what we eat? With the best intention, no doubt, you regard the matter from too low a plane. Has not the greatest of teachers himself told us that "Not that which goeth into the mouth defileth a man; but that which cometh out of the mouth, this defileth a man"?

VEGETARIAN: You know well the text has not the meaning you put on it. It could as logically be made to excuse any swinishness whatsoever. Flesh-eating is not a mere ceremonial question of eating "with unwashed hands," as that referred to in the text, but one that involves the gravest issues of right-doing and wrong-doing.

PSYCHIC PHILOSOPHER: But to the pure all things are pure.

VEGETARIAN: Possibly—if we know who *are* the pure. But the mere eating of impurities is scarcely proof sufficient.

PSYCHIC PHILOSOPHER: I cannot take your view of the importance of this question. To me, as to the Indian yogis, the choice of food is a matter of indifference.

VEGETARIAN: I doubt if your butcher's bill would bear out that assertion. If food is one of the "indifferent" things, why do you hold fast to your flesh meat, like a snarling dog to his bone?

Our psychic philosopher, in truth, is a wolf in sheep's clothing—a carnalist in psychical disguise.[33]

It will be objected, no doubt, that the injurious effect of flesh food on morals has never been scientifically proved,[34] nor indeed is it possible that absolute proof should be forthcoming until vegetarianism is widely enough practised to furnish data for comparison; there are, however, certain very marked indications that can hardly be overlooked. In the first place, as already stated, there is the immemorial belief, especially prominent in the usage of monastic orders, but scarcely less so in all systems of hygienic or spiritual exercise—amounting, in short, to a practical consensus of mankind—that a stimulating or excessive diet is harmful to sobriety and self-control; as evidenced by the far greater amount of crime rife among luxurious town-dwellers than among frugal peasants. Secondly, there is the fact, too well attested to be challenged, that flesh-eating and alcoholism are closely allied, and that the drink-crave dies a natural death when a stimulating diet is withdrawn; from which it may be further realised that the excitation caused by flesh food must necessarily, in many cases, act injuriously on the nerve-system and contribute powerfully to the vicious habits which moralists deplore.

"The deepest, truest, and most general causes of prostitution in all great cities," says Dr. Kingsford, "must be looked for in the luxurious and intemperate habits of eating and drinking prevalent among the rich and well-to-do. The chief element of this luxury is the use of flesh and alcohol, which mistaken notions of hygiene and therapeutics tend to press more and more upon all classes of men and women. Abolish kreophagy and its companion vice, alcoholism, and more, a thousandfold, will be done to abolish prostitution than can be achieved by any other means soever as long as these two evil influences flourish. The young man of the present day, accustomed from childhood to frequent and copious meals of flesh, and from early youth to the use of all manner of fermented beverages and liqueurs, carries about with him and fosters an increasingly disordered appetite, which not infrequently assumes the character of true disease."[35]

The evils of stimulating diet in the case of the young have been emphasized by such well-known authorities as Dr. George Keith and Sir B. W. Richardson. Here is a significant passage from the writings of the former:

"I have done much for many years privately, whenever I had the opportunity, to impress on fathers and mothers the danger to their sons and daughters from exciting prematurely

57

their natural desires and passions; but custom and fashion have so powerful a hold, especially in the higher circles of society, that I have frequently had to feel that my efforts were in vain.... The existence of bad habits at schools is well known to the masters, and they take what measures they can for their prevention. Even when they know the truth, the strength of custom and habit so imperatively demands a full diet for the growing youth that they are obliged to fall in with the customs of the day. But few of them are aware of the main cause of the evil, and the last thing most would dream of as a remedy is a simpler diet."[36]

So, too, Sir B. W. Richardson:

"In all my long medical career, extending over forty years, I have rarely known a case in which a child has not preferred fruit to animal food. I say it without the least prejudice, as a lesson learnt from simple experience, that the most natural diet for the young, after the natural milk diet, is fruit and wholemeal bread, with milk and water for drink. The desire for this same mode of sustenance is often continued into after years, as if the resort to flesh were a forced and artificial feeding, which required long and persistent habit to establish its permanency as a part of the system of every-day life."[37]

Contrast with this wise and weighty advice the dietetic habits actually prevalent among the youth of our well-to-do classes, where we see not only a strong tendency to over-eating, but a rooted and active conviction that flesh is the *summum bonum* of food. The fatted calf is rivalled by the fatted schoolboy; the cramming of Strasburg geese itself is not more disgusting than the cramming which makes *pâté de foie gras* of the moral fibre of the young. When we find even the *Eton College Chronicle* raising a protest against the diet of boyish athletes, we may be sure the evil is a crying one:

"He [the boy in training] takes a lot of exercise, and finds he has a good appetite. For breakfast he has a chop every morning; we have known some who had two. He also has heard porridge is nourishing, and that this is why Scotchmen are so hardy and brawny. He acts upon this information. For dinner he makes a point of having two good helpings of meat 'to get his weight up,' while for tea, besides having a plate of eggs and chicken, or something of that kind, he winds up with a large allowance of marmalade."

Nor is it only among schoolboys that over-eating is rampant, for the tables of the wealthy are everywhere loaded with flesh meat, and the example thus set is naturally followed, first in the servants' hall, and then, as far as may be, in the homes of the working classes. To consume much flesh is regarded as the sign and symbol of well-being—witness the popular English manner of keeping the festival of Christmas. "We interknit ourselves with every part of the English-speaking world," said the journal of the Cosme colony, in Paraguay, describing a Christmas celebration, "by the most sacred ceremony of over-eating." A nice moral bond of union, truly, between colonies and motherland! What is likely to be the effect on the national character of such patriotic gorging?

We come back, then, to the point that though it is not absolutely true that "man is what he eats," there is, nevertheless, a large element of truth in the saying, and the vegetarian has just ground for suspecting that beefy meals are not infrequently the precursors of beefy morals. Carnalities of one kind are apt to lead to carnalities of another, and fleshly modes of diet to fleshly modes of thought. "Good living," unfortunately, is a somewhat equivocal term.

THE ECONOMIC ARGUMENT

"The oftener we go to the vegetable world for our food," says Sir B. W. Richardson, "the oftener we go to the first, and therefore the *cheapest* source of supply." The case for vegetarianism would by no means be complete without a statement of the economic view, though precedence is necessarily given to the motives of humanity and healthfulness, the higher considerations to which the idea of economy must be subservient. If it were proved that flesh food is essential to the real interests of the race, and that there is no moral objection to the use of it, the greater outlay would be justified by the value of the result; but if such proof is not forthcoming (and it has been the object of the preceding chapters to show that it is not), it is obvious that the comparative cost of a flesh diet and a vegetarian diet becomes a question of high importance to mankind. What, then, are the facts?

They are so plain as to be positively beyond dispute, and it is a cause for marvel what Dr. J. Burney Yeo can have meant in describing vegetarianism as "a scheme of diet which we believe to be utterly impracticable on an extensive scale, and irreconcilable with the existing state of civilised man, not so much on strictly physiological grounds as *on general economical considerations*."[38] If it be in accordance with "general economical considerations" to pay threepence for what can be procured for a penny, then only does Dr. Yeo's statement become intelligible.

For the very first fact that demands notice in this comparison of foods, is that not only does butchers' meat, pound for pound, cost about three times the price of the cereals and pulses, but that it is under the further disadvantage of containing a much larger percentage of water—that is to say, in purchasing flesh, you have to buy the water, and buy it dirty, while in purchasing seeds and grains you do not buy the water, but add it clean. The following passage from Sir B. W. Richardson's "Foods for Man" puts the case succinctly:

"If we make an analysis of the primest joints of animal food, legs of mutton, sirloin of beef, rump steak, veal cutlet, pork chop, we find as much as 70 to 75 per cent. of water.... Oatmeal contains 5 or 6 per cent.; good wheaten flour, barley meal, beans and peas, 14; rice, 15; and good bread, 40 to 45 of water. Taking, then, the value of foods as estimated by their solid value, there are, it will be observed, a great many kinds of vegetable foods which are incomparably superior to animal."

We find accordingly, when we turn from this analysis to the actual charges at restaurants, that, whereas a good vegetarian dinner may be got for a shilling, it is necessary to pay fully three times that sum for an equivalent in flesh food. It would be waste of time to argue further that vegetarianism, whatever its other advantages and disadvantages to the individual, is much more *economical* than flesh-eating.[39]

But here we are met by the difficulty that the well-to-do, on the one hand, are not easily influenced by the motive of economy, while the poor, on the other hand, are naturally suspicious of the gospel of "thrift," so often preached to them by the predatory classes who do not practise it themselves; and it must be admitted that it is perfectly useless for philanthropical persons to preach food-thrift to the poor, unless by their own method of living they are testifying to the truth of what they preach.

It is sometimes said that vegetarianism is an "inconvenient" diet, which means no more than that the adoption of any new system gives trouble at first, though it may save trouble afterwards. When once adopted, vegetarianism is, of course, a far more convenient, because a simpler and cleaner diet than the ordinary one, as is testified by those who have had personal experience of both. "Having been my own butcher and scullion," says Thoreau, "as well as the gentleman from whom the dishes were served up, I can speak from an unusually complete experience. The practical objection to animal food in my case was its uncleanness, and besides, when I had caught and cleaned and cooked and eaten my fish, they seemed not to have fed me essentially. It was insignificant and unnecessary, and cost more than it came to. A little bread or a few potatoes would have done as well, with less trouble and filth."[40]

The assertion that the cheapening of food would cause the lowering of wages is true only as an answer to the exaggerated claims sometimes made by vegetarians, that their system would of itself solve the whole problem of employment. It would not do so; and if there were no force but vegetarianism in the field it is doubtful whether the adoption of the cheaper diet would in the long run bring any economical advantage to the workers, though it would still benefit them morally and physically. This, however, does not detract from the real strength of the vegetarian argument; for with labour now organised and resolute, and yearly growing in power and intelligence, there is no likelihood that the workers' thrift would become the capitalists' profit; on the contrary, it would clearly add to the resources of labour. To assert that the working classes should maintain the cruel and wasteful practice of flesh-eating merely to "keep up wages" is pure nonsense, for the same reasoning would justify the maintenance of drink, or any other extravagant and useless habit.

What is true for the individual and the class is true also for the community, and unless flesh food can be shown to be necessary for human progress, the continuance of pastoralism, to the detriment and neglect of agriculture, is a criminal waste of the national resources. In this Malthusian age of over-population scares and emigration schemes it is well to recollect that a remedy lies close to hand if we would but use it. "Not only is the earth not yet a quarter peopled," says Mr. W. R. Greg, "but even the inhabited portion is scarcely yet a quarter cultivated. In many countries the soil is barely scratched. Even in England it is not made to yield, on the average, more than one-half its capacity."[41] And in the same work he points out that "the amount of human life sustainable on a given area, and therefore throughout the chief portion of the habitable globe, may be almost indefinitely increased by a substitution *pro tanto* of vegetable for animal food.... A given acreage of wheat will feed at least *ten* times as many men as the same acreage employed in growing mutton."

In view of the great complexity of the land question, the variety of the causes that have led to the depression of agriculture, and the difficulty of forecasting accurately what would be the result of the adoption of any particular reform by any one nation, considered apart from the rest, vegetarians will do wisely in not claiming too much for the system they advocate. But at least it must be admitted that vegetarianism would tend to bring about, in some form or other, that much-desired *return to the land*, which, in the present congested state of our cities and busy centres, is felt to be the best hope of stanching a dangerous wound. The town is at present draining the life of the country, and the tide of emigration is still further sapping the national strength; but if men's thoughts could be turned back from commerce to agriculture, if a healthy love of the soil, of fruit-growing, of market-gardening, could be substituted for the insane thirst for the feverish atmosphere of the town, it is evident that a great step would have been taken towards the cure of the disease. "If the towns renounced flesh-eating," says Professor Newman, "we should see in a single generation, even without improved land-tenure, a tide of migration set the other way—from towns into the country. Rustic industry would be immensely developed. All motive for the expatriation of our robustest youth would, for a long time yet, be removed, and the country might be enormously enriched, not in an upper stratum of great fortunes, but down to the bottom of the community."[42]

So, too, Max Nordau, in some notable passages of his *Conventional Lies of our Civilisation*:

> "If the soil of Europe were cultivated like that of Belgium, it could support a population of 1,950 millions much more completely and abundantly than the 360 millions it now supports so poorly.... Cultivation of the soil is the despised child of our civilisation. It hardly takes one forward stride where manufacture takes a hundred.... Experience teaches us

that man's labour as a general thing can nowhere be employed in a more lucrative way than in agriculture. If a man should work over his field with the shovel and spade instead of the plough, he would find that a plot of ground of incredibly small size would be sufficient to support him."

There is yet another peril that would be lessened in proportion to the increase of vegetarianism—the dependence of this country on the importation of food from abroad. "At present," says Mr. W. E. A. Axon, "probably one-half of the population is dependent upon a foreign supply. That England should be, and is, the last country in the world to desire a Chinese wall for the exclusion of foreign commodities, need not blind us to the fact that there may be grave national dangers in the soil of the country providing food for about half its people. A nation of vegetarians would create such a demand that rural England would be, if not a cornfield, yet a vast orchard and market-garden."[43]

Enough has now been said to show that the habit of flesh-eating, involving as it does the sacrifice of vast tracts of land to the grazing of cattle, and the consequent starving of agriculture, is far too costly to be justified, in the face of an extending civilisation, unless by a much clearer proof of its necessity than any which its advocates have essayed; in fact, it only remains possible, on its present large scale, through the temporary use of huge pasture-grounds in remote semi-civilised regions which will not always be available. For pastoralism belongs rightly to another and earlier phase of the world's economics, and as civilisation spreads it becomes more and more an anachronism, as surely as flesh-eating, by a corresponding change, becomes an anachronism in morals.[44] It seems, generally speaking, that the foods which are the costliest in suffering are also the costliest in price, whereas the wholesome and harmless diet to which Nature points us is at once the cheapest and most humane.

DOUBTS AND DIFFICULTIES

We have next to deal with a special class of irregular foemen, the guerillas and Bashi-Bazouks of the flesh-eater's army, whose game it is to waylay and harass the vegetarian movement by a small fire of doubts and difficulties as to what the future has in store. The alarmists they are, whose apprehensive minds are concerned not so much with the rightness or wrongness of the system, as with the anxieties of "what would happen" if the triumph of vegetarianism should be won; and so gloomy are their forebodings as to suggest a probable collapse of the whole fabric of society, if once that great prop and mainstay of civilisation—the habit of eating dead animals—should be disloyally undermined.

Now, at the outset, it should be said that the well-worn method of trying to discredit new principles by "wanting to know" beforehand exactly how everything will happen, is in many cases a foolish and fraudulent device. There are, of course, certain quite legitimate questions, as to the general scope and practicability of any proposed reform, to which reformers must be prepared to make answer before they can expect to prevail, and to such questions vegetarians have a convincing reply; but when the inquisition takes the form of asking for a present explanation of future developments, and for a foreknowledge of details which, in the very nature of things, are unknowable, then it is well to make it clear from the beginning that we will be no parties to any such waste of time. Reasonable foresight is one thing, the gift of prophecy is another; and it is in no wise the duty of those who are working towards a more or less distant goal, to give a precise geometrical survey of their Promised Land.

In the case of vegetarianism the answerable doubts and difficulties fall mostly under two heads, relating first to the alarming discomforts which the loss of flesh-food would entail upon mankind, and secondly to the not less grievous straits to which the animals themselves would be reduced under so misguided a régime. Let us take the selfish view first, as containing, perhaps, a modicum of real feeling, which can scarcely be found in that suspicious concern for the animals. There are some folk, it seems, over whose troubled minds there really *does* hang, like a nightmare, the alarmist's vision of a world impoverished and dismantled by vegetarianism—a world *sans* leather, *sans* bone, *sans* soap, *sans* candles, *sans* manure, *sans* everything.

ALARMIST: But this is mere trifling. It is idle to talk of the humanity, the wholesomeness, the economy of a vegetarian diet, while you are overlooking the disastrous consequences that stare you in the face. We may perhaps be able, as you say, to exist without meat, but what could we do without leather and the other animal substances on which civilisation depends?

VEGETARIAN: Well, I suppose we should take care *not* to be without them, or something just as good.

ALARMIST: How could we do that, if there were no carcases to supply us with hides, bone, and tallow? In your devotion to an ideal you seem to forget that if your principles prevailed, we might wake up some fine morning to find ourselves confronted by the dislocation of the boot trade, the bookbinding trade, the harness trade, and a hundred others. Thousands of men and women would be thrown out of work, and we should soon have no boots, no portmanteaus, no soap, no candles, no knife-handles. It would be a downright relapse into barbarism.

VEGETARIAN: But, happily, your lurid picture is based on the false assumption that vegetarianism would come about by a sudden and instantaneous conversion. That is not the way in which great changes are accomplished. They are a matter of years and centuries, not of days and weeks; and the "fine morning" you spoke of will be a gradual morning of very extensive duration.

ALARMIST: Well, but that is only putting off the evil day—it would come at last.

VEGETARIAN: But would not something else have also been coming meantime? Would not the demand, in this as in all other usages of life, have produced the corresponding supply? There is no need, however, to speculate as to what *would* happen, because it is happening already.

ALARMIST: What is happening?

VEGETARIAN: The articles which you named are being supplied in substitutes from the vegetable kingdom. Slowly and tentatively at first, as is inevitable while vegetarians are so few in numbers; but vegetarian boots, vegetarian soap, and vegetarian candles are now in the market, and as the movement spreads, the demand will be proportionately greater. So pray do not alarm yourself about the dislocation of trade, for the whole change, great as it is, will come to pass imperceptibly, and will never bring a moment's inconvenience to anyone. Mankind, as it happens, is not so helpless, so uninventive, so literally "hidebound," as to let its progress be dependent on skins, bones, and guts.

There is a good deal of unintended humour, too, in some of the difficulties that are alleged. Thus, vegetarians are often asked how the land could be fertilised without the use of animal manure, it being apparently forgotten that *ex nihilo nihil fit*, and that animals can only return to the land in manure what they have previously taken from it in food; also that by our absurdly wasteful drainage system we are all the time poisoning our seas and rivers with a mass of sewage which would be amply sufficient for the soil. "Let the land," says Mr. William Hoyle, "only receive, in the shape of manure, the sewage and refuse from the teeming population of our towns and villages, in addition to the other means which are applied to it, and let it be properly drained and cultivated, and there is hardly any limit to its power of production."[45]

But it is superfluous to spend time in answering such questions, for their silliness is far in excess of their honesty. For years the opponents of vegetarianism in the press had been asking, "What should we do without leather?" etc.; yet as soon as the substitutes for these articles began to be exhibited at the annual Vegetarian Congress, the note was changed, and the reporters remarked that the exhibition was "not of much interest," until we found the London correspondent of a big provincial paper actually complaining that "the crusade against meat of every kind, *and even against leather* (at this exhibition they have boots and shoes made of imitation leather), is carrying the reform a little too far." Our critics are hard to satisfy. We are going "a little too far" if we produce a substitute for leather; if we do not produce one, we are not going far enough.

And now, with all becoming gravity, we turn to the second branch of our subject—the disinterested inquiry as to "what would become of the animals" if we ceased to kill them for food. "If the life of animals," says Dr. Paul Carus, "had to be regarded as sacred as human life, there can be no doubt about it that whole industries would be destroyed, and human civilisation would at once drop down to a very primitive condition. Many millions would starve, and large cities would disappear from the face of the earth. But the brute creation would suffer too. There might be a temporary increase of brute life, but certainly not of happiness. Cattle would only be raised for draught-oxen and milk-kine, and they would not die the sudden death at the hands of the butcher, but slowly of old age or by disease."[46]

A pathetic picture, indeed! It does not for a moment occur to this sapient prophet of disaster that the adoption of vegetarianism will necessarily be gradual, and further that vegetarians do *not* hold the life of animals to be "as sacred as human life." To critics who do not even ascertain what the system means before they reject it, and who ignore all consideration of the degrees and relative sacredness of the various forms of life, vegetarianism must naturally seem to be a confused jumble of thought—the confusion, in reality, being altogether on their own side.

> ALARMIST: There is another aspect of this question, and a very grave one. If flesh-eating were abolished, what would become of the animals?
>
> VEGETARIAN: Yes, let us talk about that fearful contingency. You think they would be thrown out of employment, so to speak—would find their careers cut short, or rather left long?
>
> ALARMIST: It is no joking matter. Would they not run wild in ever-increasing numbers, and perhaps overrun the land, or, if food failed them, lie dead and dying about our roadways and suburbs?
>
> VEGETARIAN: Before I relieve your anxiety on this point, may I just remark that this second difficulty seems to counterbalance the former one? If every suburban householder is likely to have a dead ox against his garden-gate, we evidently need not fear the failure of the leather and tallow trade. But once again you are mistaken. You have overlooked the fact that the breeding of animals is not free and unrestricted, but is kept within certain limits, and carefully regulated by man; so that if the demand for butchers' meat should gradually decline, there would be no more alarming result than a corresponding gradual decline in the supply from the breeder.
>
> ALARMIST: Well, I don't know. I sadly doubt whether things would balance themselves so comfortably.

VEGETARIAN: Ah, you think that some neglected old porker, like Scott's "Last Minstrel," would be left out in the cold.

"For, well-a-day! their date was fled,
His tuneful brethren all were dead;
And he, neglected and oppressed,
Longed to be with them and at rest."

But no; for look at the case of the donkey. We do not (knowingly) eat donkeys, yet a dead donkey is proverbially a rare sight. Nor are we overrun with donkeys—at least, not in the sense referred to.

ALARMIST: Yet I understand that in India, where there is a reluctance to kill animals, they are often in wretched plight.

Vegetarian: True; but we were talking not of *killing* animals but of *eating* them. Vegetarianism is not Brahminism; we would kill when necessary, whether for our own sake or the animals', but we would not breed them in vast numbers in order to kill, nor kill them in order to eat. Surely the distinction is a clear one?

The attitude of vegetarians towards this subject is indeed plain enough for those who wish to understand it. Regarding the slaughter of animals for food as cruel and unnecessary, they advocate its discontinuance (a process which, if it comes about at all, will, as I have shown, be a gradual one, and will at no point cause any sudden disruption of existing conditions), but this does not commit them to the absurd belief that animal life, in all its various grades, is absolutely sacred and inviolable. Must we not suspect that the apologists of flesh-eating who make these childish alarums and excursions are fain to do so from some inner conviction of the weakness of their own case?

BIBLE AND BEEF

"Bible and Beer" is the title that is sometimes sarcastically applied to the political alliance between churchmen and publicans; and in like manner the dietetic alliance between the "unco' guid" and the butchers may be not inaptly designated as Bible and Beef. When all else fails, the authority of Holy Writ is triumphantly cited by the bibliolatrous flesh-eater as the great court of appeal to which the food question must be carried; and here at least, it is pleaded, there can be no doubt as to the verdict. "It seems to me," wrote Dr. William Paley, more than a hundred years ago, "that it would be difficult to defend this right [to the flesh of animals] by any arguments which the light and order of Nature afford, and that we are beholden for it to the permission recorded in Scripture."[47]

It is a far cry from the theologian of 1784 to the *Meat Trades' Journal* of to-day, but from an editorial article we learn that the organ of the butchering trade is animated by the same profound sense of piety. "The great Creator of all flesh," it says, "gave us the beasts of the field, not only for our food, but for other purposes equally as essential to us. The grass must be eaten by our flocks and herds, otherwise the fertility of the soil would vanish. It was a frightful punishment on the Egyptian [*sic*] King that he should be reduced to the level of the beasts of the field and eat grass."[48]

Now, waiving the fact that grass is not precisely the diet that vegetarians adopt, and that it is, therefore, no reproach to vegetarianism if Nebuchadnezzar, not being a ruminant, found such a regimen distasteful, we must recognise that there is a widespread idea among religious people that the lower animals were "sent" us as food, and that the practice of flesh-eating has the seal of biblical sanction. In meeting this prejudice, there is a right line and a wrong line of reasoning, both of which have at different times been followed by vegetarian speakers.

The wrong line is to attempt to answer the texts quoted as favourable to flesh-eating by pitting against them other texts as favourable to vegetarianism—a course which not only degrades the Bible into a text-book for disputants,[49] but also surrenders the most sacred claim of the reformed diet—viz., its appeal not to this or to that textual authority, which some thinkers accept and others deny, but to the universal principle of humanity and justice.

The right line is to show, first, that it is wholly impossible, in the face of modern knowledge and evolutional science, to maintain the old "anthropocentric" idea which regarded man as the sum and centre of the universe, a monarch for whose special benefit all else was created; and, secondly, that the ancient Hebrew scriptures, whatever be their exact significance for Christian readers (a matter with which we are not here concerned), cannot be regarded as affording any clue to the solution of modern problems which have arisen centuries later. It would be no whit more absurd to argue that negro-slavery is justifiable because it was not condemned in the Bible than to claim scriptural sanction for the cruelties of butchery because the Jews were flesh-eaters. And, indeed, such arguments *have* been advanced by religious people in support of slavery; we read, for example, the following in John Woolman's journal: "A friend in company began to talk in support of the slave-trade, and said the negroes were understood to be the offspring of Cain, their blackness being the mark which God set upon him after he murdered Abel; that it was the design of Providence they should be slaves, as a condition proper to the race of so wicked a man as Cain was."

But it is now time to introduce the textualist in person.

TEXTUALIST: Well, sir, I understand that you advocate vegetarianism. What sort of a religion is that?

VEGETARIAN: The real sort—the sort that has to be *practised* as well as preached.

TEXTUALIST: If it is the real sort, the proof is easy. Show me the passages in the Book.

VEGETARIAN: I beg to be excused. I do not bandy texts.

TEXTUALIST: What? You can produce no verses in support of your religion? I thought vegetarians relied on what they call the "Ten Best Texts," and here I stand ready to meet them with five-and-twenty better ones.

VEGETARIAN: I am sorry to disappoint you, but I am not one of the text-quoting vegetarians. I regard all such methods of reasoning as wholly irrelevant. There is not the least doubt that the Jews were a flesh-eating people; indeed, the very idea of vegetarianism (that is, a deliberate and permanent disuse of flesh-food for moral and hygienic reasons) was wholly unknown to them. What, then, can be the use of hunting up Bible-texts which do not refer, one way or the other, to the point at issue?

TEXTUALIST: But if it was unknown and unmentioned in the Bible, what hope for vegetarianism? It perishes like all else that is unscriptural.

VEGETARIAN: The same hope as for the abolition of slavery, or any other humane cause that has had birth in our modern era. We live and learn.

TEXTUALIST: But it is written, "Rise, Peter, kill and eat." What is your answer to that?

VEGETARIAN: It needs no answer, as you will see if you study the context.

TEXTUALIST: Then you have not a single text to set against the injunction with which I confront you?

VEGETARIAN: Not one—unless it be, "Answer not a fool according to his folly."

To repel texts with texts is a futility to which vegetarians as a body have fortunately not committed themselves, because vegetarianism appeals, without reference to religion, to the common sentiment of humaneness, and numbers amongst its adherents men of every nationality and creed. If biblical vegetarians have engaged in controversy with biblical flesh-eaters, that is their own concern; and we may rest assured that the battle will be a sham one, as the firing is with blank cartridge on both sides.

Apart, however, from such irrational argument, there is a sense in which an appeal may be fairly made to the Bible, as to any other great ethnical scripture or world-literature—that is, to the spirit, as distinguished from the letter, the context as distinguished from the text. That vegetarians, preaching and practising a doctrine of love and humaneness, should quote, "Behold I have given you every herb bearing seed ... to you it shall be for meat," as indicating the ideal primitive diet, and "They shall not hurt nor destroy in all my holy mountain," as prophetic of the ideal future, is just and appropriate, for such passages, though dealing with poetry rather than fact, are far more suggestive than any textual evidence; and when we come to ask what is the spirit of the New Testament towards such instincts as that from which vegetarianism springs—the desire to increase the happiness and lessen the suffering of all sentient life—it is plain that here, at least, the vegetarian is on unassailable ground.

But the answer to the biblical flesh-eater lies still nearer at hand. For the moment any attempt is made by him to ally the modern religious spirit with the maintenance of the slaughter-house, the incongruity of his position is revealed. Take "grace before meat," for instance, and note the flat impiety of offering thanks to God over the body of a fellow-being that has been cruelly slaughtered for the sake of our "pleasures of the table." As Leigh Hunt has remarked: "It is not creditable to a thinking people that the two things they most thank God for should be eating and fighting. We say grace when we are going to cut up lamb and chicken, and when we have stuffed ourselves with both to an extent that an orang-outang would be ashamed of; and we offer up our best praises to the Creator for having blown and sabred his 'images,' our fellow-creatures, to atoms, and drenched them in blood and dirt. This is odd. Strange that we should keep our most pious transports for the lowest of our appetites and the most melancholy of our necessities; that we should never be wrought up into paroxysms of holy gratitude, but for bubble-and-squeak or a good-sized massacre!"

But why, it may be asked, if the practice of flesh-eating is such as it is here described, do "religious" people acquiesce in it? Why indeed! except that, in these personal matters of every-day life, the religionism of to-day, like the stoicism of old, has a tendency to respect the letter, but disregard the spirit of its principles. The complaint which modern vegetarianism brings against the religious flesh-eaters is that which the humaner philosophy made, centuries ago, against the carnivorous stoics:

> "Who is this censor who is so loud against the indulgence of the body and the luxuries of the kitchen? Why do they denounce pleasure as effeminate indulgence, and make so much fuss about it all? Surely it had been more logical if, while banishing from the table sweet-meats and perfumes, they had exhibited yet more indignation against the diet of blood! For as though all their philosophy merely regarded household accounts, they are simply interested in cutting down dinner expenses, so far as concerns the superfluous dainties of the table. They have no idea of deprecating what is murderous and cruel."[50]

And so is it nowadays with the champions of Bible and Beef, for, like all formalists, they sacrifice the substance of religion to the shadow, and while for ever quoting the sacred names of justice and loving-kindness, not only oppose those principles when in conflict with their own appetites, but actually base their opposition on the authority of their "scripture." It would be impossible to do the Bible a deadlier wrong than this; for whether it be "inspired" or not, it is by universal consent a great literary monument, and those who profess to reverence it most should be the last to wish to utilise it as a handbook for reactionists—a store from which to draw irrelevant quotations for obstructing the progress of reform.

THE FLESH-EATER'S KITH AND KIN

There is nothing so pleasant as the reunion of long-separated kinsfolk, and it is the cheerful duty of this chapter to exhibit the flesh-eater in what may be called his domestic relationship, to wit, his undoubted, but somewhat forgotten, connection with the cannibal and the blood-sportsman. For, disguise it as he may, he cannot altogether escape the fact that this kinship is a real one. Kreophagist and anthropophagist, butcher and amateur butcher, are but different branches of one and the same great predatory stock. The cannibal and the sportsman are the wicked uncles of the pious flesh-eater, unrespectable descendants from a common ancestry, who have failed to adapt themselves to modern requirements, and, like belated Royalists in a Commonweal, have continued to play the old privileged game when its date is over-past, an indiscretion which has caused them—the cannibal especially—to be ignored as much as possible by their more cautious relatives. We are all familiar with that chapter of "The Egoist" (the "Minor Incident showing an Hereditary Aptitude in the Use of the Knife"), in which the youthful Sir Willoughby Patterne, already an adept at "cutting," is "not at home" to his poor relation, the middle-aged unpresentable lieutenant of marines. "Considerateness dismisses him on the spot without parley." Even such is the attitude of the respectable flesh-eater towards the bloodthirsty cannibal, and in a less extent also towards the devotee of murderous "sport."

But to the student of the food question these antique types have no little interest, as a survival from an earlier and more innocent phase of flesh-eating when the old brutality was as yet untempered by the new spirit of humaneness. They exhibit kreophagy in its extreme logical form—an anachronism, no doubt, and a *reductio ad absurdum* in the present age—but at least logical, and, therefore, not to be overlooked by those who, in their hostility to food reform, are so fond of appealing to logic.

The sportsman, for instance, is an old-world barbarian born into a civilised era, a representative of the age when flesh-food could only be obtained by the chase, and he is candid enough to avow that he does his killing, not like the butcher, in order to earn a livelihood, but for the brutal reason that he *enjoys* it. "The instincts of the primeval man," it has been well said, "food-hunting, predatory, self-preserving, re-emerge in the modern: moral sanctions are disregarded, the rights of inferior races are forgotten, and the hunter feels himself, figuratively speaking, naked, savage, bloodthirsty, and unashamed."[51] A butcher he certainly is, but an amateur butcher only, for it can hardly be contended that the preserving of game increases the national food-supply, in view of the fact that pheasants, hares, and even rabbits, are sold at a price far below their actual cost of production, and are thus a direct tax on the public resources. The blood-sportsman, then, is a member of the carnivorous family by another line of descent, which has kept a touch of the rank primitive wildness even to the present day; and this one thing alone can be said in his favour, that when he butchers in sport, he at least does the butchery himself, and does not delegate the filthy task to others. He is his own slaughterman—a mere and simple savage.

Cannibalism, again, is simply flesh-eating, free from those sentimental "restrictions" which Sir Henry Thompson and his fellow scientists deplore, and the cannibal's only fault, judged from the scientist's standpoint, is that he carries out the scientific doctrine not wisely but too well. For this reason every lecture on vegetarianism ought to touch on cannibalism as illustrating a past chapter in the great history of diet—a past chapter as regards the leading and so-called civilised nations, but to this day a present and very instructive chapter in the world's remoter regions, from which we may learn certain lessons as to the feelings, arguments, and fallacies that attend the gradual process of transition from one dietetic habit to another. The flesh-eater generally affects to look on cannibalism as something monstrous and abnormal, a dreadful perversion of taste which has no connection with the civilised meat-diet on which our welfare is supposed to depend; but the real facts show that the truth is quite otherwise, and that the position of the cannibal who is being proselytised to give up his man-eating is in many ways analogous to that of the flesh-eater who is worried by the vegetarian propagandists. The glories of the old English roast beef may be instructively compared with the glories of the old African roast man.

It is amusing to observe that the kreophagist who, on the one side, regards abstinence from flesh food as an absurd delusion is equally confident that cannibalism, on the other side, is an unpardonable infamy, forgetting that many of the excuses that are made for flesh-eating might be made with as much justice for cannibalism also. "Prejudice is strange," says Professor Flinders Petrie. "A large part of mankind are cannibals, and still more, perhaps all, have been so, including our own forefathers, for Jerome describes the Atticotti, a British tribe, as preferring human flesh to that of cattle.... Does the utilitarian object? Yet one main purpose of the custom is utility; in its best and innocent forms it certainly gives the greatest happiness to the greatest number."[52] Nor can it be held that all cannibals are a specially degraded race, for Livingstone and later travellers quote well-authenticated instances to show that tribes addicted to man-eating are sometimes more advanced, mentally and physically, than those which abstain from such diet; and as to the hygienic merits of the regimen, does it not stand on record, in an old English ballad, that Richard Cœur de Lion was cured of a dangerous malady by eating a Turk's head, which was served up to him as the best substitute for pork? The kreophagist at present is able to pass unlimited censure on the cannibal, because the poor savage has not the wit to argue with the civilised man; but if, in these days of University Extension schemes, such a person as a scientific anthropophagist should ever make his appearance, who can say that the position might not be somewhat reversed?

> VEGETARIAN: Let me introduce you, gentlemen. You are blood-relations, I think, and should have much to say to each other. The Kreophagist—the Anthropophagist.

> KREOPHAGIST: Good morning, uncle. But I cannot admit the relationship if it is true that you are addicted to the atrocious habit of cannibalism.

> ANTHROPOPHAGIST: How atrocious, nephew? If you eat one kind of flesh, why should you abstain from another? Are you aware that they are chemically identical? Pig or "long pig"—where is the difference?

> KREOPHAGIST: Where is the difference? Can you ask me such a question?

> VEGETARIAN: It is uncommonly like the question you have been asking *me*!

> ANTHROPOPHAGIST: Your objection to human flesh is altogether a sentimental one. You are a food faddist. It is the universal law of nature that animals should prey on one another.

> KREOPHAGIST: It is not *my* nature to eat my fellow-beings.

> VEGETARIAN: Why, that is the very same answer that I made to *you*!

> ANTHROPOPHAGIST: And pray, what would become of our paupers, criminals, lunatics, and sick folk, if we did not eat them? Would they not grow to a great residuum and overrun the land? And the missionaries, too—are they not "sent" us as food? And what right have you to the name *omnivorous*, if you restrict your diet in this way? Why "omnivorous"?

The discontinuance of cannibalism marks, of course, an immense step in humane progress, and so long as the kreophagist does not absurdly claim that it is a *final* step, his case against the anthropophagist is a sure one; but if, while denouncing anthropophagy as a barbarism of the past, he refuses to see that flesh-eating must also, in turn, be replaced by a more humane diet, he lays himself open to a raking fire of criticism. Observe, for example, in view of the historical facts of cannibalism, the absolute helplessness of Sir Henry Thompson's position, when, as an objection to vegetarianism, he argues that "the very idea of *restricting* our resources and supplies is a step backwards, a distinct reversion to the rude and distant savagery of the past, a sign of decadence rather than of advance." It is true that mankind has, on the whole, largely extended its resources; but it is none the less true that, while it has acquired many new foods, it has abandoned certain old ones. It has advanced, in short, as already stated, by a process not of omnivorism, but of eclecticism, which implies not only acceptance, but rejection—a fact which knocks Sir Henry Thompson's reasoning to atoms.

The power which has condemned cannibalism is that growing instinct of humaneness which makes it impossible for men to prey on their fellow-beings when once recognised as such. A notable passage in one of Olive Schreiner's works may be quoted in illustration:

> "In those days, which men reck not of now, man, when he hungered, fed on the flesh of his fellow-man and found it sweet. Yet even in those days it came to pass that there was one whose head was higher than her fellows and her thought keener, and as she picked the flesh from a human skull she pondered. And so it came to pass that the next night, when men were gathered round the fire ready to eat, she stole away, and when they went to the tree where the victim was bound, they found him gone. And they cried one to another, 'She, only she, has done this, who has always said, I like not the taste of man-flesh; men are too like me: I cannot eat them.' Into the heads of certain men and women a new thought had taken root; they said, 'There is something evil in the taste of human flesh.' And ever after, when the flesh-pots were filled with man-flesh, these stood aside, and half the tribe ate human flesh and half not; then, as the years passed, none ate."[53]

A strange comment this on the Andrew Wilson formula, that we should eat "that which is likest to our own composition!" For what if we have begun to recognise that the lower animals also are related to us by a close bond of kinship? From our knowledge of the past we form our judgment of the future, and see, with Thoreau, that "it is part of the destiny of the human race, in its gradual improvement, to leave off eating animals, as surely as the savage tribes left off eating each other when they came in contact with the more civilised."[54]

VEGETARIANISM AS RELATED TO OTHER REFORMS

It is sometimes held by the champions of vegetarianism that reform of diet is the starting-point and foundation-stone of all other reform—a panacea for the ills and maladies of the world. This over-estimate on the part of a few enthusiasts of an unpopular cause is due, presumably, to a revolt from the contrary extreme of depreciation; for a little thought must show us that, in the complexity of modern life, there is no such thing as a panacea for social ailments, and that, as there is no royal road to knowledge, so there is no royal road to reform. It is impossible for vegetarianism to solve the social question, unless by alliance with various other reforms that are advancing *pari passu*—so interlocked and interdependent are all these struggles towards freedom. It has been well said that, "By humanitarians, socialists, vegetarians, anti-vivisectionists, teetotalers, land-reformers, and all such seekers of human welfare, this must be borne in mind—that each of their particular efforts is but a detail of the whole work of social regeneration, and that we cannot rightly understand and direct our own little piece of effort unless we know it, and pursue it, as part of the great whole."[55]

Still more mistaken, on the other hand, is that common prejudice against food reform which would exclude it altogether from the dignity of propagandism, and would limit it to the personal practice of individuals. "There can be no objection," says Dr. Burney Yeo, "to individuals adopting any kind of diet which they may find answer their needs and minister to their comfort; it is only when they attempt to enforce what they practise on others that they must expect to encounter rational opposition."[56] Unfortunately, we have learnt by bitter experience that *rational* opposition is the last thing we can expect to encounter—as, indeed, is made sufficiently evident by Dr. Yeo's argument. For how could individual vegetarians have ever heard of the new diet except for the propaganda? And why have vegetarians, as a body, less right than teetotalers, socialists, or any other propagandists, not to "enforce," but to *advocate* their philosophy of diet with the view of ultimately influencing public opinion? This professional attempt to class vegetarianism as an idiosyncrasy, and not a system, is as irrational as it is insincere, and what its insincerity is may be seen from the fact that, though we are told at one moment that "there can be no objection" to individual practice of the diet, yet whenever individuals do attempt to practise it, they meet with the strongest possible objection from the doctors themselves!

Thus it comes about that in this progressive age, and even among those who label themselves "progressives," vegetarianism is so frequently regarded as a mere whim and crotchet, with no practical bearing on the forward movement of to-day. It is a marvel that so many "advanced" journals, which have a good word for a host of worthy causes that are fighting an uphill battle against monopoly and injustice—social reform, land reform, law reform, prison reform, hospital reform, and a hundred more—are dumb as death, or speak only to sneer, when the subject is food reform; and thus lead their readers to suppose that, whereas on all other matters there has been a great change of feeling during the past half-century, on the one matter of diet there has been no sort of progress! Yet they might easily learn, if they made serious inquiry, that the reformed dietetics, so far from being the outcome of mere sentiment about animals, have a past record based as surely on moral and scientific reasoning as that of any cause included in the progressive programme. Vegetarianism is, in truth, *progressiveness in diet*; and for a progressive to scout such ideas as valueless and Utopian is to play the part (as far as diet is concerned) of a reactionist. What is the meaning of this strange discrepancy? It must mean, we fear, that to a large number of our social reformers the reform of other persons is a much more congenial battle cry than the reform of one's self. *Hinc illæ lacrymæ.* They call vegetarianism "impracticable" for the

74

strange reason that, unlike most *isms*, it asks them to do something individually which they know they *could* do—if they wished! It is impracticable because it does not suit them to practise it.

REFORMER: Let me entreat you; give up this fanciful scheme of vegetarianism and come and work for social reform.

VEGETARIAN: Social reform without food reform! Is not that rather a lame and lop-sided business?

REFORMER: Not at all. When we have so many things to do we must do the most important ones first.

VEGETARIAN: And what are the most important?

REFORMER: Well, there is international peace and arbitration. You will admit that our first duty is to avoid unnecessary bloodshed.

VEGETARIAN: Ah, I see! And the habit of *living* by bloodshed doesn't come within your scope!

REFORMER: Then there is the land question, and the need of relieving the congestion of our crowded cities by the revival of agriculture.

VEGETARIAN: So, of course, you can't attend to a diet-system which would bring people back to the land!

REFORMER: There is also the temperance problem—the terrible evils of the drink crave.

VEGETARIAN: Which would disappear for the most part if we left off eating flesh.

REFORMER: And the welfare of animals—for to that also I devote myself. We need some stringent legislation for the better prevention of cruelty.

VEGETARIAN: We do. But as such legislation would leave your reformers dinnerless, don't you think you should revise your dietary meantime? Your reforms are excellent, I grant you; but what of *self-reform*? Does not reform, like charity, begin at home?

REFORMER: Well, well; to everyone his taste—reform or self-reform. I prefer the former; you the latter, I suppose.

VEGETARIAN: No; that is just where you are mistaken. I prefer both at once.

Reform *and* self-reform, not reform *or* self-reform—that is the true key to the solution of the social question. The work that we can do ourselves is the most wholesome condiment for the work that we can only do through society. And here let me express the hope that, as a matter of policy, vegetarians will stand aloof from all "philanthropic" schemes of *vicarious* food reform in prisons, reformatories, and workhouses; for there is no surer way of making a principle unpopular than by forcing it on the poor and helpless, while carefully avoiding it one's self. Philanthropists, if they be philanthropists, will practise what they preach; by their practice we shall know them.

To the so-called ethical, no less than to the political, school of thought the question of vegetarianism is unwelcome, obtruding as it does on the polite wordiness of learned discussion with an issue so coarsely downright: "You are a member of an ethical society—do you live by butchery?" But the ethics of diet are the very last subject with which a cultured ethical society would concern itself, and the attitude of the modern "ethicist" towards the rights of animals is still that of the medieval schoolman. The ethicist does not wish to forego his beef and mutton, so he frames his ethics to avoid the danger of such mishap, and while he talks of high themes with the serene wisdom of a philosopher the slaughter-houses continue to run blood. We surmise that the royal founder and archetype of ethical societies was that learned but futile monarch referred to in the epitaph:

Here lies our mutton-loving king,
Whose word no man relies on:
He never *said* a foolish thing,
And never *did* a wise one.

So, too, throughout the whole field of hygiene, temperance, and plain living, to ignore vegetarianism is to ignore one of the most potent influences for self-restraint. One is reluctant to quote the late Sir Henry Thompson in any matter that tends to the praise of vegetarianism, in view of the extreme irritability which that distinguished scientist exhibited as regards his sacred text, with which you could never take the liberty of assuming that, when it distinctly said one thing, it did not mean the opposite; yet he *did* say that "a proportion amounting at least to more than one-half of the disease which embitters the middle and latter part of life, among the middle and upper classes of the population, is due to avoidable errors in diet."[57] If this be so, it is obvious that diet reform (of some sort) is very urgently needed; and I submit that it would be difficult to frame any intelligible scheme of diet reform in which vegetarian principles should play no part, embracing, as they do, all the best features of temperance and frugality. What is the use of for ever preaching about the avoidance of luxuries and stimulants, if you rule out of your system the one dietary which makes stimulants and luxuries impossible? The relation of vegetarianism to temperance, of the food question to the drink question, is that of the greater which includes the less.

But it is when we turn from philanthropy to zoophily, and to the questions more particularly affecting the welfare of animals, that the importance of vegetarianism, in spite of the stubborn attempts of the old-fashioned "animal lovers" to overlook it, is most marked. Here, again, I do not share the extreme vegetarian view that food reform is the *foundation* of other reforms, for I think it can be shown that all cruelties to animals, whether inflicted in the interests of the dinner-table, the laboratory, the hunting-field, or any other institution, are the outcome of one and the same error—the blindness which can see no unity and kinship, but only difference and division, between the human and the non-human race. This blindness it is—this crass denial of a common origin, a common nature, a common structure, and common pleasures and pains—that has alone hardened men in all ages of the world, civilised or barbarous, to inflict such fiendish outrages on their harmless fellow-beings; and to remove this blindness we need, it seems to me, a deeper and more radical remedy than the reform of sport, or of physiological methods, or even of diet alone. The only real cure for the evil is the growing sense that the lower animals are closely akin to us, and have rights.

And here we see the inevitable logic of vegetarianism, if our belief in the rights of animals is ever to quit the stage of theory and enter the stage of fact; for just as there can be no human rights where there is slavery, so there can be no animal rights where there is eating of flesh. "To keep a man, slave or servant," says Edward Carpenter, "for your own advantage merely, to keep an animal that you may *eat* it, is a lie; you cannot look that man or animal in the face." I am not saying that it is not a good thing that, quite apart from food reform, anti-vivisectionists should be denouncing the doings of "the scientific inquisition," while humanitarians of another school are exposing the horrors of sport, for cruelty is a many-headed monster, and there must at times be a concentration of energy on a particular spot; but I do say that any reasoned principle of kindness to animals which leaves vegetarianism outside its scope is, in the very nature of things, foredoomed to failure.[58]

Vegetarianism is an essential part of any true zoophily, and the reason why it is not more generally recognised as such is the same as that which excludes it from the plan of the progressive—that it is so upsetting to the every-day habits of the average man. Few of us, comparatively, care to murder birds in "sport," and still fewer to cut up living animals in the supposed interests of "science," but we have all been taught to regard flesh food as a necessity, and it is a matter, at first, of some effort and self-denial to rid ourselves of complicity in butchering. Herein is at once the strength and the weakness of the case for vegetarianism—the strength as regards its logic, and the weakness as regards its unpopularity—that it makes more direct personal demand on the earnestness of its believers than other forms of zoophily do; for which reason there is a widespread, though perhaps unconscious, tendency among zoophilists to evade it.

Yet that such evasion is a blunder may be seen from the outcry raised against it not by vegetarians only, but by the vivisectionists and sportsmen themselves, who are quick to ask the zoophilists why, if they are so eager for the well-being of the animals, they do not desist from eating them—a question which, however insincere in the mouths of some who propound it, must at least be allowed to be logical. For it is simple truth that though vivisection is a more refined and diabolical torture, and sport a more stupidly wanton one, the *sum* of suffering that results from the practice of flesh-eating is greater and more disastrous than either, and by being so familiarly paraded in our streets is a cause of wider demoralisation. When one thinks of the aimless and stunted life, as well as the barbarous death, of the wretched victims of the slaughter-house, bred as they are for no better purpose than to be unnaturally fattened for the table, it makes one marvel that so many kindly folk, keenly sensitive to the cruelties inflicted elsewhere, should be utterly deaf and blind to the doings of their family butcher. The zoophilist loves to quote the famous lines of Coleridge:

> He prayeth best who loveth best
> All things both great and small.

But what kind of "love" is that which eats the object of its affection? There are hidden rocks in that poetical passage which a sense of humour should indicate to the pilot of zoophily.

Our position, therefore, is this—that while we make no exaggerated claim for vegetarianism, as in itself a panacea for human ills and animal sufferings, we insist on the rational view that reform of diet is an indispensable branch of social organisation, and that it is idle to talk of recognising "rights of animals" so long as we unconcernedly *eat* them. Vegetarianism is no more and no less than an essential part in the highly complex engine which is to shape the fabric of a new social structure, an engine which will not work if a single screw be missing. The part without the whole is undeniably powerless; but so also, as it happens, is the whole without the part.

CONCLUSION

The chief object of this work, as stated at the outset, has been to prove the logical soundness of vegetarian principles, and the hollowness of the hackneyed taunt, so often a makeshift for reasoning, that vegetarians are a crew of mild brainless enthusiasts whose "hearts are better than their heads." How far I have been successful in this purpose it is for the reader to judge; I trust it has, at least, been made plain that, if it is logic that our friends are in need of, we are quite ready to accommodate them, and that nothing will please us better than a thorough intellectual sifting of the whole problem of diet. Only it must be a *thorough* sifting. The great foe of vegetarianism, as of every other reform, is habit—that inert, blind, dogged force which time called into being, and time only can outwear—and it is this which lurks behind the flimsy sophisms and excuses that the flesh-eater loves to set up, in which, as a rule, though there is much show of controversy, there is little real discussion. To those of our opponents who honestly wish to grapple with the question of diet, and to understand what vegetarianism means (whether they agree with it or not), I submit that the following points have, at any rate, been clearly set before them:

> 1. That the objections raised to the name "vegetarian" are founded on sheer ignorance of the word's origin, and calculated, if not designed, to distract attention from the substance by fixing it on the shadow. It is not nowadays seriously denied, by any responsible authority, that a vegetable diet, *with the addition of eggs and milk*, is quite adequate for nutriment; but the method is this—to allow what is said (rightly or wrongly) of the sufficiency of a

strictly vegetable diet to be misunderstood by the public as referring to "vegetarianism." Thus, Dr. J. Burney Yeo, in his "Food in Health and Disease," first argues that "vegetarians" have no right to their title, because they consume animal products, and then proceeds to allege various reasons against "a purely vegetable diet," which by his own showing is not what vegetarianism represents. This is a fair sample of flesh-eaters' logic.

2. That the immediate aim of vegetarians is not that which, under various forms, is so industriously foisted on them—viz., a desire to attain at one step to the millennium, by altogether ceasing to take the life of animals, or by entire abstinence from animal products—but rather it is a practical, intelligible, though necessarily imperfect, attempt to humanise, as far as may be, the present sanguinary diet system, by the omission at least of its more loathsome and barbarous features.

3. That vegetarianism, if once admitted to be practicable, offers certain positive benefits of the utmost value, humane, æsthetic, hygienic, social, economic; while, on the other hand, the denials that have hitherto been made of its practicability, on the plea of structure, laws of nature, climate, digestion, and so forth, are far too weak and illogical to bear the test of criticism. There *may*, of course, be some conclusive reason against vegetarianism, but if so, why is its production delayed?

4. That in the greater number of the arguments brought against vegetarianism, the importance of the *moral* aspect of the question is studiously kept out of sight. Thus, Sir Henry Thompson, in his *Nineteenth Century* article of 1885, while admitting the possibility of abstaining from flesh foods, gave judgment on the whole in favour of a moderate use of them—but without allowing the smallest weight to humane or moral considerations. Writing on the same subject in 1898, he so far repaired this oversight as to argue that it is really kinder to eat animals than not to do so, because otherwise they would not be bred at all! That is the amount of attention the moral side of vegetarianism receives from its opponents, a great humane issue being set aside by a sophism more suited for a Savoy comedy than for serious discussion.

But there is the further question—and as far as these chapters are concerned, the final question why, if vegetarianism is part and parcel of a genuine "progressive" movement, does it not more rapidly progress? "Why so little *result* from your propaganda?" is the frequent sneer of the flesh-eater, and the vegetarian himself is sometimes fain to be down-hearted at the seeming slowness of his advance. Does vegetarianism progress? Yes and no, according to the expectations, reasonable or unreasonable, that its supporters have been cherishing. If we have fondly hoped to witness, in the future, the triumph of the humaner living, it must be allowed that the actual rate of progress is extremely disheartening; but if, on the contrary, we work under a rational understanding that a widespread change of diet, like any other radical change, is a matter not of years but of centuries, then we shall not find in the slow growth of our movement any reason for dissatisfaction. Revolution in personal habits, be it remembered, is even more difficult than revolution in political forms, and needs a greater time for its fulfilment, and, looked at in this light, vegetarianism has made as much progress during the past half-century as any other cause which aims at so far-reaching a change.

But what of the many individual failures, it is asked, among those who make trial of vegetarianism? Taking the circumstances into account, the failures cannot be regarded as numerous; for in every such movement there are half-hearted people who are impelled by motives of restlessness and curiosity, rather than of real conviction, and in view of the personal obstacles that beset the path of the vegetarian it is not surprising that in food reform, as in drink reform, there are a certain number of backsliders. In an ordinary household every possible influence, social and domestic, is brought to bear on the heretic who abstains from flesh foods. Anxious relatives and indignant friends adjure him to remember the duty he owes to himself and to his family, and urge him for the sake of those dear to him, if not for his own, to return to that great sacramental bond of union between man and man—the eating of our non-human fellow-beings. Is he smitten by one of the numberless ailments that are the stock-in-trade of the physician, and of which flesh-eaters are daily the victims in every part of the world? The doctor looks wise, shakes his head, and informs a sorrowing circle that it is the direct result of "his vegetarianism." Above all, the fear of ridicule, acting on the natural unwillingness of mankind to venture along unknown paths, is a strong deterrent; for there are still many persons to whom the idea of abstinence from butchers' meat is positively a matter for merriment, and it seems fated that vegetarianism, like every new principle, must be a target for such shafts. Well, so be it! We know that the struggle will be a long one, and if vegetarianism has got to run the blockade of Noodledom, and a huge amount of foolish talk must perforce be fired off, the sooner the battle commences, and the sooner it is concluded, the better for all concerned. And ridicule, as the flesh-eater will learn, is a weapon which can be wielded by more parties than one.

For, to be frank, the dietists of the old-fashioned kreophagist school have talked, and are talking, a great deal of downright nonsense in their tirades against vegetarianism, and the only reason why they have not been more widely brought to book is that they speak in orthodox quarters where no reply is permitted. The oracle, of course, must not be answered or criticised. So far as they have condescended to state a case against food reform, it is a case which would be laughed out of court, as a string of quibbles and absurdities, in any open discussion; for the specialist, that most humourless of persons, is apt to forget that the moment he quits the ground on which he has made himself a master (and such ground has very narrow limitations) he is no longer infallible, and that if he thinks to exorcise modern feeling by the repetition of ancient formulas, he will only make himself ridiculous. And as a matter of pure humour, apart from humanity, which is the more comical—the man who can live in simple affluence on a supply of food which is as little costly to himself as it is burdensome to others, or he who cannot be content unless he gluts an ogreish appetite on animals slaughtered for his larder, and then pharisaically pretends that he has done them a kindness by eating them? It is custom, and custom alone—the thraldom of that "ceaseless round of mutton and beef to which the dead level of civilisation reduces us"[59]— that prevents civilised men from seeing the essential silliness of maintaining the diet of savages.

That a percentage of those who make trial of vegetarianism should return to their former habit is in accordance with what always happens in the fight between the new and the old, and at the utmost—that is, in the rare cases where such trial has been a genuine one—proves only that a change of diet is much more difficult for some persons than it is for others, a fact which all rational food reformers have recognised. But from the force of *affirmative* testimony there is no escape, when, as in the case of vegetarianism successfully practised, and yielding the best results, the instances are drawn from every rank and temperament, and are amply sufficient in number to prove the experience trustworthy. It is idle to go on asserting that a thing cannot be done, when you are face to face with some thousands of people who not only have done it, but are happier and healthier in consequence.

With the question of the right choice of food, and how to adopt vegetarianism, I am not here concerned; such information is readily accessible in current vegetarian literature. But it must be said in conclusion—and this is the thought which, above all others, I would leave in the mind of the reader—that the surest warrant of success in the reform of diet is a sincere belief in the moral rightness of the cause. The *spirit* in which one takes up vegetarianism is the main factor in the result. It is useless to look for any absolute proof in such matters—the proof is in one's self—for those, at least, who have heart to feel, and brain to ponder, the cruelty and folly of flesh-eating. It is an issue where logic is as wholly on the one side as habit is wholly on the other, and where habit is as certainly the shield of barbarism as logic is the sword of humaneness.

FOOTNOTES

1. *Nineteenth Century*, May, 1885.

2. *Ibid.*, June, 1898.

3. As in "The Perfect Way in Diet," by Dr. Anna Kingsford; and "Strength and Diet," by the Hon. R. Russell.

4. See the list of names cited in Mr. Howard Williams's "Ethics of Diet," a biographical history of the literature of humane dietetics from the earliest period to the present day.

5. "Odontography," chap. x., p. 471, 1840-1845. This sentence is quoted only for what it is worth—viz., as proving that, in Owen's opinion, man was originally frugivorous. If the whole passage in "Odontography" be studied, it will be seen that Owen cannot fairly be cited as a vegetarian authority, because, after alluding to the fact that the apes occasionally eat insects, eggs, and young birds, he sums up in favour of what he calls "the frugivorous and mixed regimen of the quadrumana and man." This point I have dealt with later in the chapter.

6. "Foods for Man," *Longman's Magazine*, 1888.

7. It has been well shown by Dr. J. Oldfield, in the *New Century Review*, October 1898, that "omnivorism" in the hoggish sense, is *not* characteristic of progressive mankind. "The higher we go in the scale of life, the more we find *selection* taking the place of omnivorism. The more complex the organism, the greater its selective capacity. 'Selection,' then, rather than 'omnivorism,' should be the watch-cry of the human race evolving upward."

8. *Humane Science Lectures*: Summary of address given by Prince Kropotkin at Essex Hall, November 17, 1896.

9. "Study of Animal Life."

10. "Evolutional Ethics and Animal Psychology."

11. Wollaston, "Religion of Nature," 1759.

12. December 29, 1898.

13. *Fortnightly Review*, November, 1895.

14. The *Ethical World*, May 7, 1898.

15. *Ibid.*

16. *Fortnightly Review*, November, 1895.

17. *Illustrated London News*, May 14, 1898.

18. "Behind the Scenes in Slaughter-houses."

19. *Daily Telegraph*, July 19, 1897.

20. *New Age*, November 25, 1897.

21. From a series of letters contributed to the *Nottingham Guardian* by Mr. J. F. Fraser, author of "America at Work."

22. See the official facts and figures cited in "Tuberculosis," by Dr. J. Oldfield, 1892.

23. *Reynolds's Newspaper*, March 19, 1899.

24. The "Author's Case."

25. "Uric Acid as a Factor in the Causation of Disease. Diet and Foods Considered in Relation to Strength and Power of Endurance."

26. *British Medical Journal*, June 4, 1898.

27. "Foods of Man."

28. Rees's "Encyclopædia," Article, "Man."

29. *Vegetarian Messenger*, January, 1899.

30. *Nineteenth Century*, August, 1898.

31. Edward Carpenter, "The Art of Creation," "Health a Conquest."

32. Walden, "Higher Laws."

33. It is a curious fact that the Greek word *psychic* had the double sense of *spiritual* and *carnal*. See Tertullian's treatise, "Against the Carnal-Minded" (Psychicos).

34. Even cannibalism—such is the complexity of the human character—is not always *directly* demoralising. "This unnatural practice," says Captain Burrows in his "Land of the Pigmies," 1899, "stands by itself, seeming not in any way to affect or retard the development of the better emotions."

35. "The Perfect Way in Diet."

36. "Fads of an Old Physician," chap. xiv.

37. "Foods for Man."

38. "Food in Health and Disease."

39. See the chapter on "Values of Foods," pp. 93, 94, in "Strength and Diet," by the Hon. R. Russell.

40. Walden, "Higher Laws."

41. Appendix to "Enigmas of Life."

42. "Essays on Diet," p. 55.

43. *Manchester Vegetarian Lectures*, "Vegetarianism and National Economy." For a clear statement of the present shocking neglect of agriculture in this country, see "Fields, Factories, and Workshops," by P. Kropotkin, 1899, where it is shown that *two-thirds* of our food-supply is now imported from abroad.

44. Against the sea fisheries, it may be noted, the same objection cannot be raised, as they do not diminish, but supplement the produce of the soil.

45. "Our National Resources," 1889.

46. "The Open Court," 1898.

47. "Moral and Political Philosophy."

48. November 19, 1892.

49. As in the epigram,

Hic liber est in quo quærit sua dogmata quisque,

Invenit et pariter dogmata quisque sua:

which may be freely rendered,

This is the Book, to dogmatists well-known,

Where each man dogma seeks, and finds—his own.

50. Plutarch, "On Flesh-Eating," quoted in "The Ethics of Diet," by Howard Williams.

51. Robert Buchanan. Preface to J. Connell's "The Truth about the Game Laws."

52. For interesting facts concerning cannibalism, see Professor W. M. Flinders Petrie's article, *Contemporary Review*, June 1897; "The Fall of the Congo Arabs," by Captain Sidney L. Hinde, 1897; and "The Land of the Pigmies," by Captain Guy Burrows, 1899.

53. "Trooper Peter Halket."

54. Walden, "Higher Laws."

55. The *New Charter*, "The Humanitarian View."

56. "Foods in Health and Disease."

57. *Nineteenth Century*, May, 1885.

58. Take, for example, the rule to which some bird-lovers bind themselves, to wear no feathers but those of birds killed for food. One is reminded of Thomas Paine's epigram: "They pity the plumage, but forget the dying bird."

59. Richard Jefferies, "Field and Hedgerows."